FROM MIASMAS TO MOLECULES

Number 13

BAMPTON LECTURES IN AMERICA

Delivered at Columbia University

1961

FROM MIASMAS

NEW YORK AND LONDON 1961

TO MOLECULES

W. BARRY WOOD, JR., M.D.

COLUMBIA UNIVERSITY PRESS

PREFACE

THE FOUR ESSAYS which comprise this book concern the progress of medical science. They deal with a single disease, selected for discussion because it is probably the most successfully studied illness known to man. The story of its conquest admirably illustrates the manner in which the applications of natural science have revolutionized the practice of medicine and public health.

The purpose of relating this story in the Bampton Lectures of 1961 was not to extol the accomplishments of modern hygiene; rather, it was to introduce an element of historical perspective into current discussions of the social shortcomings of modern medicine and to document the conclusion that the principal problems which plague the medical profession today are the inevitable consequences of scientific progress.

ACKNOWLEDGMENTS

THE FOLLOWING JOURNALS and publishers have graciously granted permission to reprint illustrations:

Yale Journal of Biology and Medicine (Figs. 1, 2, 3)
Lucien Mazenod, Geneva (Figs. 4, 6)
W. B. Saunders Company, Philadelphia (Fig. 13a)
The C. V. Mosby Company, St. Louis (Fig. 10)
Cambridge University Press (Fig. 11)
Annals of the New York Academy of Sciences (Fig. 12)
Merck Report (Figs. 13b, 13c)
Journal of General Physiology (Figs. 14a, 14b)
John Wiley & Sons, Inc., New York (Figs. 14c, 15, 16)
Journal of Molecular Biology (Fig. 14d)
Springer-Verlag (Fig. 18)
Scientific American (Fig. 21)
New York *Times* (Figs. 23, 24, 25)

I wish to thank Dr. Oswei Temkin, Professor of the History of Medicine of the Johns Hopkins University, and Dr. Edwards A. Park, Emeritus Professor of Pediatrics, for their helpful criticisms of the original manuscripts, and Miss Concetta Loiero and Mrs. Nancy Gruber for their many typings of the text. Finally, I would like to express to Columbia University my deep appreciation of the invitation to serve as a Bampton Lecturer.

CONTENTS

FIGURES

MIASMAS

Let's search the Cause, 'tis breach of Laws,
    That punishes for Sin,
That brings down Plagues in every Age,
    as it has ever been.

A LAMENTATION

IN THE YEAR 1706 the senior class of Yale College was composed of three students. In keeping with the primary purposes of the institution, all three became ministers of the gospel. One of them, Jonathan Dickinson, was promptly called to the church at Elizabeth Town, New Jersey, and in 1747 he was appointed the first president of the College of New Jersey, which later became Princeton University.[1]

Dickinson, one of the most influential religious leaders in the colonies, was also of necessity a physician. Few trained doctors were available in America before 1750, and the heavy burden of caring for the sick and the dying often fell upon the clergy. Besides many religious pamphlets, which gained him widespread fame among his contemporaries, he wrote a medical work of the first order entitled *Observations on that terrible Disease vulgarly called the Throat Distemper with advices as to the Method of Cure*.[2]

"This Distemper," Dickinson related, "began in these Parts, in February, 1735. The long Continuance and universal Spread of it among us, has given me abundant Opportunity to be acquainted with it in all its Forms.

"The first Assault was in a Family about ten Miles from me, which proved fatal to eight of the Children in about a Fortnight. Being called to visit the distressed Family, I found upon my arrival, one of the Children newly dead, which gave me the Advantage of a Dissection, and thereby a better Acquaintance with the Nature of the Disease, than I could otherwise have had."

Not all minister-physicians of his day would have had the urge to perform an autopsy on such an occasion, but, as the following passage indicates, Dickinson was a meticulous and discerning student of disease.

"It frequently begins," he wrote of the throat distemper, "with a slight Indisposition, much resembling an ordinary Cold, with a listless Habit, a slow and scarce discernable Fever, some soreness of the Throat and Tumefaction of the Tonsils: and perhaps a running of the Nose, the Countenance pale, and the eyes dull and heavy. The patient is not confined, nor any Danger apprehended for some Days, till the Fever gradually increases, the whole Throat, and sometimes the Roof of the Mouth and Nostrils are covered with a cankerous Crust. . . . When the lungs are thus affected, the Patient is first afflicted with a dry hollow Cough, which is quickly succeeded with an extraordinary Hoarseness and total Loss of the Voice, with the most distressing asthmatic Symptoms and difficulty of Breathing, under which the poor miserable creature struggles, until

released by a perfect Suffocation, or Stoppage of the Breath.
This last has been the fatal Symptom, under which the
most have sunk, that have died in these parts. And indeed
there have been few recovered whose Lungs have been

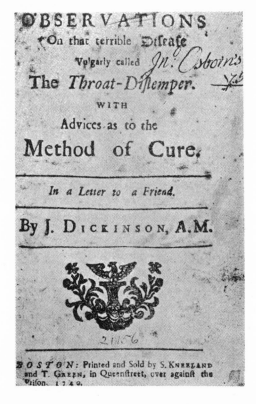

*Figure 1. Title page of Dickinson's treatise on
throat distemper*

(Reprinted from E. Caulfield, *The Throat Distemper of
1735–1740*, New Haven, Yale Journal of Biology and Medicine,
1939.)

thus affected. All that I have seen get over this dreadful Symptom . . . have by their perpetual Cough expectorated incredible Quantities of a tough whitish slough from their Lungs, for a considerable Time together. And on the other Hand, I have seen large Pieces of the Crust, several inches Long and near an Inch broad, torn from the Lungs by the vehemence of the Cough. . . . "

Such a detailed clinical description could only have been written by one who had spent countless hours caring for patients with this dreadful malady.

In the same year that Dickinson observed his first case in New Jersey, a similar epidemic broke out in far-off Kingston, New Hampshire.[1] Ten years earlier the Reverend Ward Clark had been called to be the first minister of the town, which was inhabited by only eighty-one families. He had been a schoolteacher at nearby Exeter and had received a master's degree at Harvard in 1723. Beloved by his congregation, he became the natural leader of the community. During the first decade of his ministry sickness was rare, and the population doubled. What illness there was he treated as best he could, for there was no doctor in Kingston.

In 1735, spring came late to New Hampshire; the weather was unusually wet and cold. On May 20, Parker Morgan, the son of John Morgan, suddenly died after a brief illness. A week later, in a house on the other side of the town, more than four miles away, the three children of Jeremiah Webster died within three days. News of the tragedy which had struck the Webster family rapidly spread through the

community. All three children seemed to have suffered
the same illness which had taken Parker Morgan. Yet the
families lived miles apart and had not mingled for months.
There was something strange about this sickness.

In the month that followed there were more deaths in
Kingston than usually occurred in a whole year. Each was
briefly mentioned by the distraught Clark in the parish
records: [3]

June y^e   5 Deborrah Child of Joseph Batchelor Died
           7 Dorothy Daughter of Jacob Gilman Died
          17 Samuel Loch Lost a Daughter
          18 Ebenezer Sluper Lost a son. Both died with a Quincey
          19 Samuel Emons Eldest Daughter Died
          21 Died David son of Joseph Greely
          23 Samuel Emons lost another
          23 The Same Day Ebenezer Sluper Lost another
          25 Andrew Webster Lost his Child
          25 Joseph Bean lost one of His Children
          27 Died another of Joseph Bean's Children
          28 Died Margaret Eldest Daughter of Joseph Bean
          30 Samuel Emons Lost another Child.

So ended the sorrowful account of the month of June.
But the raging epidemic had just begun. In July, nineteen
more succumbed, including Clark's wife and youngest
child. In August, two more of the Clark children died, and,
by the end of December, the death toll had reached the
unprecedented figure of 102. For the next three years the
epidemic continued. On August 29, 1736, Clark lost his
only remaining child. Having ministered to the best of
his ability to his afflicted congregation and having lost his
beloved wife and all of his four children, Clark finally
could endure no more. In the spring of 1737, he returned

to Exeter and died a few months later. By the end of 1738, the dreaded sickness had visited nearly every family in the community, and more than a third of all the children in the town had died. Of the first forty who were taken ill not a single one recovered.

Concerning the nature of the strange "Plague in the Throat," which decimated his people, Clark left only the following brief statement in the church record: "This Mortality was By a Kanker Quinsey or Peripn (eumony), which mostly seized upon young People and has Proved Exceeding mortal in Several other Towns y^t It is supposed there never was ye like Before in this Country." According to later historical accounts, many of the stricken children died within twelve hours, some of them expiring without any apparent respiratory distress, "while sitting up at play with their playthings in their hands." [4]

From Kingston the epidemic spread rapidly to neighboring towns in New Hampshire [5] and on eastward to the small coastal communities of Maine.[6] At the same time it moved southward into Massachusetts along the main road from Hampton to Boston.[7] Once it had crossed the Merrimac River, the Boston selectmen became alarmed and called together the most distinguished physicians of the city and its suburbs to advise them as to ways and means of protecting the public. Among those summoned was Dr. Simon Tufts of Medford, whose large practice extended into the northern townships already invaded by the epidemic. Having had personal experience with the disease, he explained to his colleagues the strange ways of the "Eastern Distemper": how it first appeared mysteriously in Kingston in two homes four miles apart; how it spread

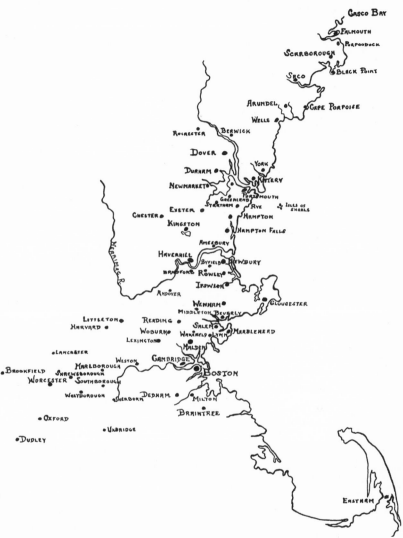

Figure 2. Map of coastal communities of New England colonies in 1735

(Reprinted from E. Caulfield, *The Throat Distemper of 1735–1740*, New Haven, Yale Journal of Biology and Medicine, 1939.)

from one New Hampshire town to another without any apparent contacts between the inhabitants; how its ravages failed to be controlled by the conventional medical treatment of the day; and how few of those afflicted were able to survive more than a short time. Upon hearing his account and discussing in full all that was then known of the illness, Dr. Tufts's colleagues could reach only one important conclusion: "the said Distemper was communicated by means of a bad Air and not by Contagion." Shortly thereafter the disease made its appearance in Boston, and before the epidemic had subsided, it had involved about a fourth of the people. Though the mortality was lower in Boston, there is little doubt that the disease was the same as that which occurred in New Hampshire. The difference in mortality was, of course, attributed by the Boston doctors to their professional superiority over the practitioners and ministers of the smaller rural communities.

Meanwhile, in Connecticut another epidemic began, not in the regions close to Massachusetts but in the extreme southwest corner of the colony, at Stamford. The following reference to the new outbreak appeared in the Boston *News-Letter* of February 19–26, 1736:

"We have an Account from Connecticut, that the Distemper that has for some Months past prevail'd at the Eastward, has now got into the Western Part of that colony, where several Children and Young People have lately died; particularly at Stamford, where one Mr. John Smith has buried Five Children in a little more than a Fortnight; and some Families in that Town that had but Three or Four Children have buried them all." [8]

Two features of the Connecticut epidemic are of particular interest. First, as shown in the accompanying map (Fig. 3), it gradually spread eastward from Stamford and

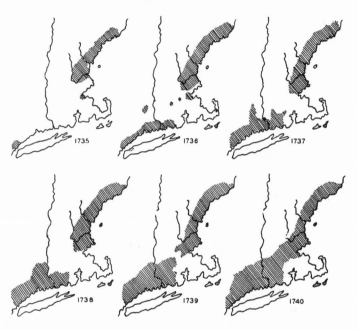

Figure 3. Map showing spread of epidemics of throat distemper in New Hampshire and Connecticut between 1735 and 1740

(Reprinted from E. Caulfield, *The Throat Distemper of 1735–1740*, New Haven, Yale Journal of Biology and Medicine, 1939.)

did not enter Massachusetts from the south until late in 1739. The direction of its spread strongly suggests that it originated from a focus separable from the New Hampshire-Massachusetts epidemic, possibly in New Jersey.

Second, the Connecticut epidemic was milder than the New Hampshire one. The case fatality rates were five times lower in Connecticut, and multiple deaths in individual families were less frequent. Thus, the two epidemics differed not only in origin but also in severity.

To the devout colonists the coming of the "throat distemper" was an act of God—the "Fruit of strange Sins." To be sure, contagion was recognized in the case of smallpox; indeed, most provinces had strict laws designed to prevent its spread. In Rhode Island, for example, the penalty for violating the rules of smallpox sanitation was death "without benefit of clergy." But the "throat distemper" had begun in two widely separated parts of Kingston, and its spread from town to town appeared to follow no understandable pattern. Sudden outbreaks arising in relatively isolated communities, where no one had previously been ill, soon led to the conviction that the disease was spread not by contact but by miasmas or, as the Boston physicians had concluded, by "bad air." And the "bad air" came as a warning to the people from an angry God. In the words of the pastor at the North Church in Portsmouth:

"The Progress of the late Distemper has been very strange in its passing from one Town to another, after a considerable space of Time, and in its long remaining in one Part of a Town, before it has passed into other parts, and in its returning when it seemed to be quite gone, and the Fears of it were blown over; on these Accounts the Act of Providence is the more visible in sending it, and

we are led to look beyond natural Causes to the Hand of
God, to whom we are chiefly concern'd to apply our selves
for the removal of this awful Calamity." [9]

How awful the calamity was is not hard to imagine
if we recall the public panic wrought by the far milder
epidemics of our own experience—epidemics of poliomye-
litis and of influenza. What is more difficult for us to
appreciate is the abysmal deficiencies in medical knowledge
which existed in the early eighteenth century. The serious
handicaps of ignorance which beset the doctors of colonial
America are vividly illustrated by the general theories of
contagion prevailing in 1735.

According to medical historians, the first signs of an
appreciation that disease may be communicated by contact
is found in the recorded customs of the early Jews and
Egyptians. The book of Leviticus in the Old Testament
contains the following familiar reference:

"And the leper in whom the plague is, his clothes shall
be rent, and his head bare, and he shall put a covering upon
his upper lip, and shall cry Unclean, unclean. All the days
wherein the plague shall be in him he shall be defiled; he
is unclean: he shall dwell alone; without the camp shall
his habitation be." [10]

The concept of contagion held by the ancient Jews was
virtually abandoned in the Greek and Roman period, primarily because of the teachings of Hippocrates. According
to the Hippocratic doctrine, all pestilence was due to
cosmo-telluric phenomena: eclipses, earthquakes, floods,
and, in particular, pollution of the air by miasmas. Indeed,

bad air containing poisonous miasmas, derived from smelly swamps and putrefying animal matter, was claimed to be the principal cause of illness.[11] This theory, expounded also by Galen, remained predominant until the Middle Ages when the idea of contagion was revived by such writers as Giovanni Boccaccio, who, in his famous *Decameron*, described the devastating Florentine plague of 1348. He told of the swellings in the groins and the armpits of the patients and referred to the disease as a contagion. "To touch their clothes," he wrote, "or whatever other object had been used by those who had been ill caused the communication of the disease."

Two centuries later the poet and philosopher Girolamo Fracastoro—better known by his Latinized name, Fracastorius—wrote a remarkable book based upon his own extensive studies of plague, typhus, syphilis, and foot-and-mouth disease in northern Italy. He defined contagion as an infection which passes from one individual to another. He spoke of three types of contagion: (1) contagion by contact alone; (2) contagion by fomites; and (3) contagion at a distance. "I call fomites," he wrote, "clothes, wooden things and other things of that sort which in themselves are not corrupted but are able to preserve the original germs of the contagion and to give rise to its transference to others."[12] He even referred to the "seeds" or "germs" of disease, although his description of their nature was vague and he looked upon their action as analogous to the exhalation of an onion in causing the shedding of tears.

Although the writings of Fracastorious had an influence upon contemporary scholars, his teachings were insufficiently heeded. When the Great Plague descended on London in 1665, thousands fled the doomed city. William Boghurst, an apothecary, remained behind to offer what help he could to the terrified populace. Despite his evident

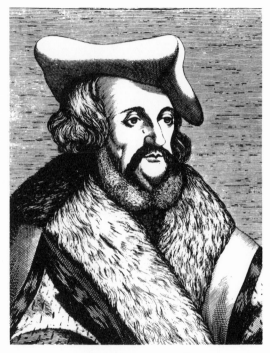

Figure 4. Fracastorius
(Reprinted from Les Médecins Célèbres, Edition d'Art, Geneva, Lucien Mazenod, 1947.)

erudition and his vast experience in the epidemic itself, he could do no better than attribute the cause of the plague to "a most subtle, peculiar, insinuating, venomous, deleterious exhalation arising from the maturation of the ferment of the faeces of the earth extracted in the aire by the heat of the sun and difflated from place to place by the winds and most tymes gradually but sometimes immediately aggressing apt bodyes." [13] Such reasoning was less sophisticated than the contagion theory of Fracastorius; nevertheless, it represented the accepted thinking of the day.

But even as the Great Plague ravaged London, a new scientific discovery was in the offing, one destined to reveal for the first time the true nature of contagion. It was made, not by a student of disease, but by a student of optics—a grinder of lenses.

Anthony van Leeuwenhoek was born in Delft, Holland, in 1632. A draper by trade, he spent his spare time making lenses and mounting them to form microscopes. This new kind of instrument had been invented by others several decades earlier, but had not been perfected. Leeuwenhoek fashioned more perfect lenses and began turning them on all manner of tiny objects. Each new finding he meticulously recorded in the voluminous diary which he wrote each day in painstaking longhand. From time to time he reported his observations in long letters to the Royal Society in London. In his now famous eighteenth letter, dated 9 October 1676, he described four sorts of minute living creatures he had observed in rain water. "The fourth sort of animalcules, which I saw moving about," he wrote, "were so small that, for all of me, no shape can be specified. These animalcules were more than a thousand times smaller than the eye of a full-grown louse; for I judge the diameter of the louse's eye to be more than ten times the diameter of the said creature. They exceed in speed the previously described animalcules. I have at various times seen them stopping at one point, and whirling themselves at a speed such as we see in a spinning top before our eye; and then again motion in a circle, the circumference of which was hardly greater than that of a small sand-grain; and then again either straight out or in a crooked path." [14]

Although these tiny creatures may well have been protozoa, there is no doubt that the organisms described in his thirty-ninth letter, of 17 September 1683, were bacteria. These he obtained from around his own teeth. Some were apparently motionless, others had "a very strong and swift motion and shot through the water (or spittle) like a pike does through water." Their varied morphologies are clearly recognizable today as those of the coccal, bacillary, and spiral species of bacteria which commonly inhabit the mouth.

Thus the marvelous world of microbes was first revealed to man. But, as is so often the case with revolutionary discoveries, the true significance of Leeuwenhoek's observations was not realized for many generations. There is no suggestion in his own writing that any of these tiny animalcules might be related to the cause of human illness. Nor was this thought advanced by others more familiar with medicine, with an occasional notable exception.

In 1720 there was published in London a remarkable book entitled *A New Theory of Consumptions: More Especially of a Phthisis or Consumption of the Lungs*. It was written by Benjamin Marten, an obscure practitioner who lived in Theobald's Row. Concerning the etiology

of consumption (now, of course, known as tuberculosis)
Marten advanced the following hypothesis:

"The Original and Essential Cause, then, which some
content themselves to call a serious Disposition of the Juices,

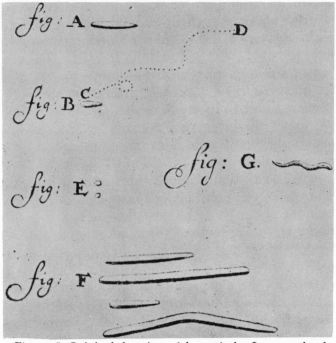

Figure 5. Original drawing of bacteria by Leeuwenhoek
(Reproduced from *Arcana Naturae delecta ab Antonio van
Leeuwenhoek*, Delphis Batavorum apud Henricum Crooneveld,
1695.)

others a Salt Acrimony, others a strange Ferment, others
a Malignant Humour, may possibly be some certain Species
of *Animalculae* or wonderfully minute living creatures
that, by their peculiar Shape or disagreeable Parts are in-

imicable to our Nature; but, however, capable of subsisting in our Juices and Vessels."

As to the contagiousness of the disease he suggested that "The minute Animals or their Seed . . . are for the most part either conveyed from Parents to their Offspring hereditarily or communicated immediately from Distempered Persons to sound ones who are very conversant with them. . . . It may, therefore, be very likely," he continues, "that by an habitual lying in the same Bed with a consumptive Patient, constantly eating or drinking with him or by very frequent conversing so nearly as to draw in part of the Breath he emits from the Lungs, a Consumption may be caught by a sound Person . . . . I imagine that slightly conversing with consumptive Patients is seldom or never sufficient to catch the Disease, there being but few if any of these minute Creatures . . . communicated in slender conversation." [15]

Marten predicted that his theory would be more acceptable to those who were aware of the invisible world of microscopic animalcules than to those who had no idea of living creatures "besides what are conspicuous to the bare eye." Manifestly his whole thesis was based on Leeuwenhoek's discoveries. One hundred and sixty years later it was proved by Robert Koch to be essentially correct. But at the time it aroused no interest whatsoever, for the medical profession of Marten's day was unreceptive to the theory of contagion. As a result his book was soon forgotten. When in 1911 it was rediscovered, only four copies, and very little information about the author, could be found.

The low regard in which Leeuwenhoek's animalcules were held by scientists in general is suggested by the manner in which Linnaeus, who was himself a physician, classified them in the 1767 edition of his *Systema Naturae*. Placing them under "Vermes," in a class which he designated "Chaos," he grouped them with "the ethereal clouds suspended in the sky in the month of blossoming." [16]

Such was the climate of medical science when the "throat distemper" struck the American colonies in 1735. No wonder the doctors and ministers of New England and New Jersey were baffled by this terrible affliction which ravaged their towns and villages. To them it was an entirely new disease, for they did not know that Spanish and Italian writers had described it a century earlier. Of Marten's theory of contagion they were either ignorant or skeptical.

To be sure, Cotton Mather, dead only seven years, had had a microscope.[17] In a sermon delivered in Boston in 1689 and entitled "The Wonderful Work of God Commemorated: a Thanksgiving Sermon," he had referred to the microscopic marvels which he himself had seen:

"And the *Little* things which our Naked Eyes cannot penetrate into, have in them a Greatness not to be seen without Astonishment. By the Assistance of *Microscopes* have I seen Animals of which many hundreds would not Equal a Grain of Sand. How Exquisite, How stupendous must the Structure of them be! The Whales . . . methinks . . . are not such Wonders, as these minute Fishes are." Coming even from Cotton Mather (who was apparently familiar with the work of both Marten and Leeuwenhoek), these statements had no influence on colonial medicine.

His fire-and-brimstone theology had taught the colonists to seek a religious interpretation of every event of their daily lives and to accept adversity as a just punishment for sin. Since science could not explain epidemics, they were accepted by all as acts of God. The afflicted people turned to the church for help, and there they found the spiritual strength to bear what befell them.

The throat distemper, which wrought havoc in His Majesty's Colonies, was not a new disease. Knowledge of its existence appears to date back to Hippocrates in the fourth century B.C.[18] Aretaeus, the Cappadocian, described it in the second century A.D. and, believing that it had come from Egypt and Syria, termed it the Egyptian or Syriac ulcer.[19] Perhaps the best early description is that of Aetius, the personal physician of the Emperor Justinian, who lived in the sixth century. Writing on "pestilential lesions of the tonsils," he stated:

"They occur most frequently in children, but also in adults . . . . Usually in children the evils known as aphthae develop. These are white, like blotches; some are ashen in colour or like eschars from the cautery. The patient suffers from a dryness of the gullet and frequent attacks of choking . . . . A spreading sore supervenes in the region afflicted . . . . In some cases the uvula is eaten up and when the sores have prevailed a long time and deepened, a cicatrix forms over them and the patient's speech becomes rather husky and, in drinking, liquid is diverted upward to the nostrils. I have known a girl to die even after forty days when already on the way to recovery." [20]

During the dark ages, medical writings were scanty, and there were few additional references to the disease until the murderous epidemics which swept the Spanish peninsula in the sixteenth and seventeenth centuries.[21] Because one form of the distressing illness frequently led to suffocation, the Spaniards called it *morbres suffocares* or the *garrotillo*.[22] The connotation of the latter term is appreciated only by those who know its derivation from the word *garrot*, which means a stick or lever. Its use was suggested by the barbaric custom of slowly strangling criminals to death by looping ropes about their necks and gradually twisting them tight with garrotes. So many children died of the disease in 1613 that the year became known in Spanish history as "the year of the *garrotillo*."

In the century that followed, similar epidemics occurred in other parts of Europe. In Italy and Sicily the affliction was known as the "gullet disease." [18] In 1625, Cortesius of Messina recorded the remarkable case of the Warden of St. Francis, who, suffering from a severe inflammation of the throat, complained of a foul breath. To make sure that he was not merely imagining the bad odor, he asked a friend to smell the exhalations from his mouth. Shortly thereafter the friend came down with the illness and died of suffocation on the fourth day. "From this instance," wrote Cortesius, "I have come to the conclusion that the disease is more or less contagious." [23]

With such lucid descriptions as these already set down in detail by European physicians, why were the doctors of New England unaware of them in 1735? The answer is no doubt to be found in the limited distribution of

medical writings in this period and the relative isolation
of British medicine from that of the Continent. There is
documentary evidence that few doctors in England had
recognized the disease prior to the colonial outbreak. In
1739 a London apothecary, baffled by strange cases of
"putrid sore throat" which occurred in his neighborhood,
called in consultation a "very learned and sagacious" Dr.
Letherland, who, much to the amazement of all, identified
the affliction as the Spanish *garatillo*.[24] With the disease
thus virtually unknown in London, it is not surprising that
news of it had not reached the colonies.

In the years that followed, further confusion was engendered by the writings of Francis Home of Edinburgh.[25]
In 1765 he published *An Inquiry into the Nature, Cause
and Cure of Croup*, which he considered to be a totally
new and rare disease. Several of the cases he described were
clearly cases of throat distemper, but because of the exalted
position he held as physician to the King, his terminology
became widely accepted both in England and abroad. When
in 1807 the nephew of Napoleon Bonaparte died of throat
distemper, the Emperor, although campaigning in Prussia
at the time, immediately gave orders for an open competi-
tion and offered a prize of 12,000 francs for the best scientific essay on the croup.[18] The results of this contest, though
it lasted for over five years, did little to clarify the situation.
But fourteen years later, in 1826, a publication appeared
which started a new era in medicine.

Among the physicians who attended the child Napoléon
Louis Charles during his fatal illness was Pierre Fidèle
Bretonneau—the physician in chief of the General Hospital

at Tours. Having studied in great detail a sizable epidemic of throat distemper which occurred in and about Tours in 1819, he concluded that the outbreak was due to a specific disease, characterized by the formation of a false

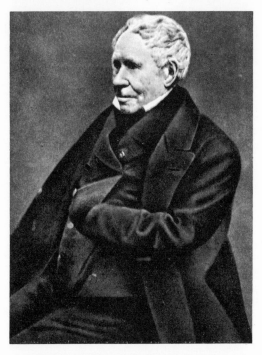

Figure 6. Pierre Fidèle Bretonneau
(Reprinted from Les Médecins Célèbres, Edition d'Art, Geneva, Lucien Mazenod, 1947.)

membrane in the respiratory tract. Because of the membrane, which clearly differentiated it from other afflictions of the throat, Bretonneau called the malady *diphtheritis*, derived from the Greek word meaning skin or membrane.

Later the designation was changed to *diphtheria*, the term by which the disease is known today.

On June 26, 1821, Bretonneau communicated his findings to the Académie Royale de Médecine, and in 1826 he published them in an extensive monograph, now considered one of the great classics of clinical medicine.[26] His shrewd observations led him to the conviction that diphtheria is a communicable disease, transmitted from person to person, and caused by a specific germ, which in turn is responsible for the characteristic membrane. His views on etiology were, of course, entirely speculative, for the science of bacteriology was still unborn.

MICROBES

Antitoxin and antibacterial substances are, so to speak, charmed
  bullets which strike only those objects for whose destruction
  they have been produced. PAUL EHRLICH

PIERRE BRETONNEAU's recognition of diphtheria as a clinical
entity, separable from other inflammations of the throat,
was not his greatest contribution to medicine. Rather it
was his proposal of the general theory that different diseases
are due to different specific causes.[1] This doctrine of etio-
logical specificity, first enunciated in the 1820s, is now
so firmly established that it is hard for us to imagine how
it could ever have been doubted. Yet its acceptance by
the medical profession was extremely slow, partly because
Bretonneau's own writings did not make it sufficiently
clear. Not until the closing decades of the nineteenth
century did it finally become recognized as a cardinal
principle of clinical medicine.

Interestingly enough, its first confirmation came in the
1830s from an amateur scientist, Agostino Bassi of Italy.
A Doctor of Laws, he had attended a few scientific lectures
early in his life at the University of Pavia. Although primarily a civil servant and often on the verge of poverty,

he became so interested in a disease of silkworms, known as *calcino*, that he devoted nearly twenty years of his life to the study of its cause.

The pestilence received its name because, after death, the affected worms became covered with a white coating of lime-like consistency. The origin of the affliction was completely unknown. By persistent efforts, which were said to have cost him his eyesight, Bassi proved that the disease was caused by a specific contagion.[2] Although the characteristic white coating appeared only after death, he showed that individual worms were infective at much earlier stages. By first searing their outer skins in a flame, then pricking their bodies with a preheated pin, he successfully transferred the malady to healthy silkworms. Later, despite his defective eyesight, he identified microscopically the parasitic fungus which caused the infection. In the closing years of his life, when increasing blindness precluded further microscopy, he wrote extensively on the application of his contagion theory to human disease.[3] In the case of cholera, for example, he advocated immediate isolation of the patient and disinfection of the clothes and excreta. Thus, Agostino Bassi became the founder of the doctrine of parasitic microbes.

Bassi's views on cholera were dramatically amplified in the same period by John Snow, an anesthetist of London.[4] His classic epidemiological observations were made not with a microscope but "with a notebook, a map and his five senses." During the London cholera outbreak of 1854, Snow noted that in the region of Lambeth Palace and Southwark Cathedral, on the south bank of the Thames, there were two separate water supplies. That from the Lambeth Company served 26,000 houses and came from the Thames at a point relatively free of human pollution. The other, from the Southwark Vauxhall Company, was used by more than 40,000 houses and was taken from the Thames at Battersea Fields, where there was ample opportunity for sewage contamination. During the first seven weeks of the epidemic, according to Snow's figures, 300 patients died—286 of them in houses supplied by the Southwark Vauxhall Company and only 14 in the ones supplied by its competitor. But this was only the beginning of Snow's laborious study. Shortly thereafter, a relatively isolated epidemic erupted in Broad Street. More than 500 deaths occurred in ten days within 250 yards of the house where the outbreak began. By the mere process of questioning, Snow learned that practically all the deaths occurred among those who obtained water from the Broad Street pump. In contrast, there were only 5 deaths among the 535 inhabitants of a neighboring workhouse which secured its water from another source. In the Broad Street brewery, where the 70 workers apparently preferred the company's ale to water from the pump, there was not a single fatality. And most conclusive of all was the case of a well-to-do lady who had moved to Hempstead before the start of the epidemic but who had become so fond of the water from the pump that she had had a large bottle of it brought by cart each day to her new home in the country. She and the niece visiting her both died of the cholera. Snow's conclusion was obvious: the pump water, which he found to be contaminated with organic matter, was the source of the malignant disease. When he finally persuaded the Board of Guardians to have the handle removed from the fatal pump, the epidemic promptly subsided.

No less convincing were the similar studies of William Budd on the relation of contaminated water to typhoid fever [5] and the famous observations of Oliver Wendell Holmes [6] in America and of Ignaz Semmelweis [7] in Vienna, both of whom concluded that childbed fever was transmitted from patient to patient by the unclean hands and the contaminated clothing of the attending obstetrician. Despite the mounting evidence advanced in its support, however, the germ theory of disease was fiercely opposed by the medical profession. The open hostility it engendered is vividly exemplified by the behavior of Semmelweis's colleagues, whose violent reactions were in keeping with an age when dogma was passed down uncritically from generation to generation and empiricism prevailed. Much of this rigidity of thought was to change, for a new science was about to emerge—the science of bacteriology, or, as it is now called, microbiology.

Following Bassi's discovery of the silkworm fungus, pathologists began to look diligently for other microbes in the diseased tissues of man. New methods of staining were developed, and many previously unknown microorganisms were described. Often more than one kind of tiny animalcule was found in the same specimen. What, if anything, did these minute creatures have to do with the patient's illness? This became the critical question to which the pathologists had no answer.

In the case of diphtheria, numerous attempts were made to transfer the disease to other human subjects and to laboratory animals, just as Bassi had transmitted the calcino to healthy silkworms. Though the human tests failed, probably because of immunity factors, a few of the animal experiments met with success. The most impressive were those performed in Munich by Oertel at the close of the Franco-Prussian War.[8, 9] First, he produced false membranes in rabbits by swabbing their throats with membranous exudates obtained from human cases of diphtheria. And then, to prove that the rabbit lesions were not caused by some inanimate irritant or merely by the trauma of the swabbing procedure, he attempted to produce them in series. Having infected rabbit 1 with human exudate, he inoculated rabbit 2 with purulent matter taken from the resulting lesion in rabbit 1; then, as soon as rabbit 2 had developed a suitable lesion, he took from it a sample of exudate, which he inoculated into rabbit 3, and so on. In one instance he passed the experimental disease through a series of six rabbits, and, much to his satisfaction, the sixth one developed a false membrane resembling that seen in human diphtheria. Clearly, he was dealing with a living agent which was capable of multiplying in the tissues of normal rabbits. Was this the specific germ of diphtheria or was it some other infective agent which merely happened to be present in the original human exudate? This critical question remained unanswered by Oertel's experiments. Its importance lay in the fact that human diphtheritic membranes, when carefully examined under the microscope, were usually found to contain more than one kind of microbe. Several different yeasts and molds had been identified in the membranes and each had been designated the cause of the disease.

Such was the state of confusion when the Congress for Internal Medicine met in Wiesbaden in 1883. One of the topics discussed at this historic meeting was diphtheria. The principal speaker on its etiology was the irascible German pathologist Edwin Klebs, of Zurich, who had studied with the great Virchow. While a professor at Prague, in 1875, he described a specific fungus in human diphtheritic membranes which he had named *Microsporon diphtheriticum* because he was certain that it caused the disease.[10] At the Wiesbaden Congress he astonished the audience by asserting that the diphtheria he had observed in Zurich was entirely different from that which he had studied in Prague.[11] The new variety, he claimed, was produced by a bacillus which, when stained with methylene blue, appeared to have a knob at either end. It was always present on the surface of the local membranes, but never could be found in other tissues of diphtheria victims. These findings forced him to conclude that there were at least two kinds of diphtheria, one caused by a fungus, the other by a bacillus. But because of his congenital impatience Klebs failed to follow up his discovery of the bacillus, and the etiology of diphtheria remained in doubt.

Meanwhile a Prussian army surgeon, Friedrich Löffler, was at work in the laboratory of Robert Koch, who the year before had gained immortal fame by discovering the cause of tuberculosis.[12] Koch had devised a method of growing bacteria in pure culture.[13] This he had done by adding solidifying agents, such as gelatin, to nutrient media in which the organism was known to grow. When a sufficiently dilute suspension of a mixture of different kinds of bacteria was properly spread over the surface of the

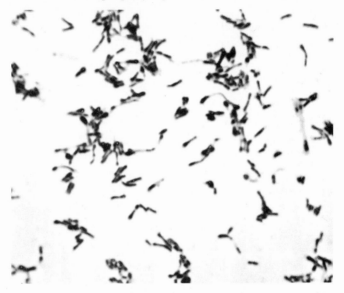

Figure 7. Klebs-Löffler bacilli stained with methylene blue

solid medium, each organism thus inoculated eventually grew into a discrete colony composed solely of its own progeny. Since each kind of bacterium formed a characteristic colony, one species was easily differentiated from another. Pure cultures of each species in the original mixture could then be obtained from subcultures made from each type of colony. Koch's discovery of this relatively simple method revolutionized the study of infectious disease, for it enabled pathologists, for the first time, to work with

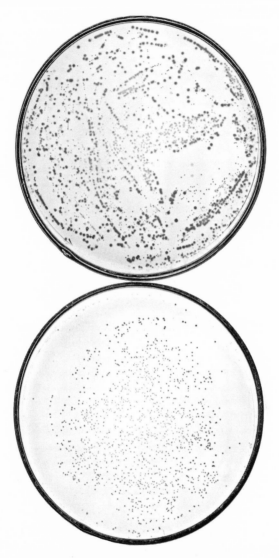

Figure 8. Mixed (top) and pure (bottom) cultures of bacteria growing in discrete colonies on surface of solid medium contained in Petri plates

single microbial species rather than with heterogeneous mixtures. This, and much more, Löffler learned from his masterful teacher.

In undertaking the study of diphtheria, Löffler was well aware of the pitfalls which lay before him.[14] That diphtheria was a single malady caused by a specific infectious agent, he was relatively certain. But he knew also that the throats of diphtheria patients harbored many microorganisms other than the germ of the disease. How could he separate the one responsible microbe from this conglomerate mixture, and how could he prove its causative role?

As a first step he made a detailed microscopic study of tissues recovered from twenty-seven fatal cases of inflammation of the throat. Twenty-two of the patients were thought to have had diphtheria; the remaining five, "scarlatinal diphtheria." The latter designation was used whenever the rash of scarlet fever accompanied the inflammation of the throat. Although many clinicians at the time considered the scarlatinal form to be a variant of so-called pure diphtheria, others believed it to be a distinctly different disease. The issue was clearly settled by Löffler's systematic observations. For in the scarlatinal group he found that the dominant microbe in the respiratory tract was a micrococcus, which tended to form chains. It had been described nine years earlier in septic wounds and in a severe skin infection known as erysipelas. Because of its chain-forming property it had been given the name streptococcus. Besides being present in the throat, where they appeared to have produced deep necrotic lesions very different from the superficial membranes of diphtheria, the streptococci were also found in the deep lymphatic vessels of the neck, in the blood stream, and in various internal tissues located at considerable distances from the original infection of the

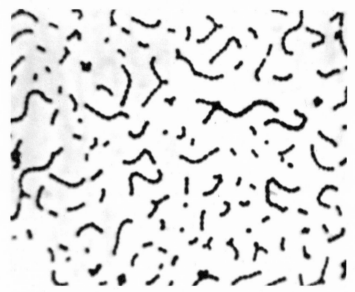

Figure 9. Streptococci of the type Löffler found in throats of patients dying of "scarlatinal diphtheria"

tonsils. The internal spread of the microbes, Löffler concluded, had been caused by an invasion of the general circulation, known as septicemia.

In the larger group of cases, which had been diagnosed as pure diphtheria, streptococci were also found in the throat but in smaller numbers. Their presence in the typical superficial membranes was overshadowed by another organism which Löffler quickly recognized as the Klebs bacillus. It stained properly with methylene blue and was easily demonstrable in thirteen of the twenty-two cases. Unlike the streptococci in the scarlatinal cases, the Klebs bacilli were situated only in the outermost layers of the false membranes, where they often appeared in a relatively pure state, unmixed with other microorganisms. Never did they penetrate the deeper tissues of the throat or invade the blood stream; and, despite the most careful search, they were never found in any of the internal organs. As to the eight cases in which he failed to find the Klebs bacillus, Löffler tentatively concluded that it might originally have been present and might somehow have been eliminated before death. But obviously his evidence was still flimsy.

Next he set to work to culture the two organisms from the tissues. The streptococci were easily grown on Koch's peptone-gelatin medium, and pure cultures were obtained by the plating technique already described. Heavy suspensions of the cultured streptococci were then inoculated into mice, rabbits, guinea pigs, pigeons, fowl, canaries, a dog, and a monkey. Although most of the animals became ill and a number died of generalized infections, in no case did inoculation of the throat result in a disease which resembled human diphtheria.

Isolation of the Klebs bacillus, on the other hand, turned out to be much more difficult for an interesting reason. Because gelatin plates liquify above 24° C., they can be used only to culture organisms which will multiply at relatively low temperatures. Whereas streptococci grow reasonably well at these low temperatures, Klebs bacilli do not. There-

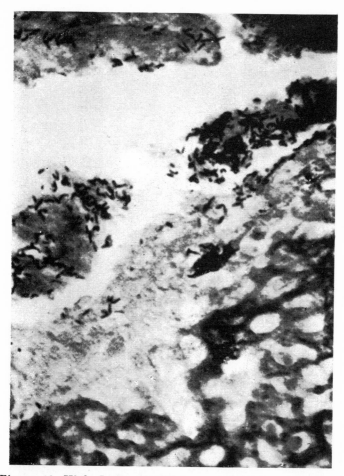

Figure 10. Klebs-Löffler bacilli in superficial layer of pharyngeal membrane from fatal case of diphtheria. The thin section of membrane overlying throat tissue was treated with a special "bacterial stain" designed to reveal the microbes lodged within the exudate

(Reprinted from W. A. D. Anderson, *Pathology*, St. Louis, The C. V. Mosby Company, 1957.)

fore, Löffler was forced to design a new type of solid medium which could be incubated at body temperature. This he did by using heated blood serum as the solidifying agent instead of gelatin. When he inoculated the new medium with membranous exudate containing a mixture of Klebs bacilli and streptococci, both organisms grew at body temperature. Since each produced a characteristic colony, he was soon able to grow the Klebs bacilli in pure cultures. These he used to inoculate laboratory animals, just as he had done with the streptococci. Whereas mice and rats were immune, guinea pigs were found to be highly susceptible. When twenty-three of them were inoculated with Klebs bacilli under the skin, they all died within two to five days. The lesions at the site of inoculation were hemorrhagic and contained many bacilli. Careful study of other tissues revealed dense brownish lesions in the lungs and marked congestion of blood vessels, particularly in the kidneys and adrenal glands. But none of these secondary lesions contained any bacilli! This remarkable fact made a profound impression upon Löffler. Indeed it forced him to conclude that the bacilli growing at the primary site of infection must have produced a soluble poison, which was transported throughout the body by the blood stream. The significance of this conjecture will become apparent presently.

Using the same cultures, he next inoculated the throats of rabbits and pigeons. In a number of instances, false membranes, which simulated those seen in human diphtheria, formed in the pharynx and trachea.

Finally, to test further his conclusion that diphtheria

was caused by the Klebs bacillus, he attempted to culture it from the throats of twenty apparently healthy children. Much to his amazement, one of the cultures was positive, and the organism isolated proved to be virulent for guinea pigs. Thus it was discovered that healthy members of a community may be "carriers" of pathogenic diphtheria bacilli.

The results of Löffler's extensive experiments were published in 1884.[14] From them he cautiously concluded that the Klebs bacillus was probably the long-sought germ of diphtheria. In discussing his findings, however, he objectively reviewed all the negative evidence as well as the positive and ended by emphasizing the urgent need for further work on the problem. His observations were soon confirmed by others, and today he is considered the principal discoverer of the cause of diphtheria.

Among those who confirmed Löffler's classic experiments were two French bacteriologists, Emile Roux and Alexandre Yersin.[15] Working at the newly founded Pasteur Institute in Paris, they demonstrated that rabbits which survived the initial stages of experimental diphtheria often developed paralysis. This finding was of great significance because paralyses were known to occur frequently in human diphtheria. Clinicians had long realized that the nervous system was often involved, particularly in the later stages of the illness. Paralysis of the muscles of the soft palate was especially common and accounted for the characteristic nasal voice and the regurgitation of fluids through the nose. Eye muscles and muscles used in swallowing were frequently affected. In more severe cases, the paralyses involved the arms, the legs, and sometimes the diaphragm and other muscles of respiration. These late neurological symptoms were, of course, well known to Löffler; indeed, he had been much disturbed that he had been unable to detect convincing signs of neuritis * in any of his infected animals. Thus, the observations of Roux and Yersin appeared to have filled an important gap in the otherwise conclusive evidence.

Having confirmed Löffler's observation that the bacilli were present only at the primary site of infection, Roux and Yersin next endeavored to isolate the postulated poison.[16] This they did by growing a pure culture of diphtheria bacilli in a suitable broth medium for a week or more, in the hope that the bacilli would release their toxin into the surrounding fluid. Then, to get rid of the living bacilli, they forced the culture through a filter of fine unglazed porcelain. The clear filtrate contained no bacteria, but, when it was injected into animals, it caused all of the manifestations produced by the living culture except the false membranes. If administered in small doses, it frequently caused paralysis; in large doses it was lethal. Its action was identical to that of the poison which could be demonstrated in the tissues and urine of diphtheria victims. Here, then, was absolute proof that the Klebs bacillus was the cause of diphtheria. Furthermore, its pathogenicity appeared to be due to two distinct properties:

* Although three of his infected pigeons had developed abnormal gaits, he was never convinced that their difficulty in walking was due to diphtheritic neuritis.

first, its ability to multiply locally in the surface tissues of the respiratory tract, where it caused the formation of a characteristic false membrane; and, second, its production of a soluble toxin, which was rapidly carried by the blood stream to other organs of the body, where it caused additional damage.

The next development, the most important of all, followed immediately. Though it stemmed indirectly from the work of Roux and Yersin, it came not from the Pasteur Institute but, once again, from Koch's laboratory. There another Prussian army surgeon, Emil Behring, was collaborating with two of Koch's assistants, Carl Fraenkel and Shibasaburo Kitasato. The latter, a Japanese bacteriologist, had just cultivated the tetanus bacillus.[17] It too had been found to produce a soluble toxin, which caused the horrible symptoms of lockjaw. Behring and his colleagues believed that there might be a way to create artificial immunities to both diphtheria and tetanus, just as Pasteur had done several years before for rabies, chicken cholera, and anthrax. The key to Pasteur's success had been the use of attenuated vaccines, which contained germs of greatly depressed virulence and therefore could be injected with relative impunity. Accordingly, Behring's group set out to develop similar vaccines.

By growing originally virulent diphtheria bacilli in nutrient broth for approximately three weeks and then heating the broth culture at a temperature of 60–70° C. for one hour, Fraenkel was able to prepare an attenuated diphtheria vaccine. When guinea pigs were injected subcutaneously with the vaccine and were challenged ten days later with a lethal dose of virulent diphtheria bacilli, they all survived. This encouraging result was reported by Fraenkel in a Berlin medical journal on December 3, 1890.[18] On the following day there appeared in the *Deutsche medizinische Wochenschrift* a related report by Behring and Kitasato.[19] It dealt with immunity to lockjaw and contained the startling statement that the blood serum of animals previously injected with appropriately prepared tetanus cultures could render the tetanus toxin innocuous. Although the authors used the word "anti-toxic" only in a brief footnote, the term "antitoxin" was eventually adopted to indicate the toxin-destroying property of the immune serum. On December 11, in the same journal, Behring himself announced the discovery of diphtheria antitoxin.[20] In this paper, the third to appear in eight days, he reported that the serum of animals immunized with diphtheria vaccine was capable of nullifying the harmful effects of diphtheria toxin.

Within a year all of these facts had been confirmed in other laboratories, and in Berlin on Christmas night, 1891, the first diphtheritic child to receive antitoxin was treated.[21] Soon the commercial production of antitoxin was begun, and large-scale clinical trials of the new serum were instituted. In one such test, which lasted a full year, a large hospital divided its diphtheria patients into two groups: those admitted on one day were treated with antitoxin, those admitted the following day were treated without antitoxin, and so on.[22] Of the 239 patients who received the antitoxin therapy, 3.5 percent died; among the

245 control cases there was a fatality rate of over 12 percent. The statistics recorded in other hospitals showed a
similar trend, and by the end of the 1890s diphtheria antitoxin had become an accepted agent of therapy.

Although generally effective, Behring's serum did not
always cure the children who received it.[23] In some cases
it was given too late; for when the toxin had had time to
act, its harmful effects could not be reversed. In other cases
the amount given was insufficient to combine with all of
the toxin produced by the organism in the throat. Sometimes death resulted not from the toxin but rather from
an obstruction of the airways by the false membrane, and
occasionally the serum itself caused serious reactions which
necessitated discontinuance of treatment. Only when treatment was instituted relatively early was the serum consistently effective.

The evident limitations of antitoxin therapy, however,
led to still another approach to the conquest of the disease.
It, too, came from Behring's laboratory, but only after
years of persistent investigation. Knowing that guinea pigs
could be made immune to diphtheria by vaccination with
Fraenkel's attenuated cultures, and knowing also that these
cultures contained soluble toxin as well as bacilli, Behring
and his collaborators tried using the toxin alone instead of
whole cultures as the immunizing agent.[20] Though the
immunity produced seemed just as impressive as that stimulated by the whole cultures, the injections of the toxin
caused severe reactions in the skin. If the toxin could only
be modified so as not to cause such reactions, it might

then be used to immunize human subjects. But how could this be done?

A satisfactory answer was first suggested in 1909 by Theobald Smith in America.[24] By this time it had been learned that the protective action of diphtheria antiserum was due to specific protein molecules called antibodies. These antibody molecules combined with the diphtheria toxin, nullifying its harmful effect. They were not present in the serum of unimmunized animals, but made their appearance only after either infection or immunization. Their action was highly specific: diphtheria antibodies combined only with diphtheria toxin, tetanus antibodies only with tetanus toxin, and so on. The specific substances which stimulated their production became known as *antigens*. Thus, the antigen responsible for the formation of diphtheria antitoxin was the diphtheria toxin itself.

In addition to the antigen-antibody concept, a second important principle relating to the distinction between *active* and *passive* immunity had been established. This distinction may be explained as follows: When an animal is made immune by the injection of serum from a second animal which has been previously inoculated with the antigen, the first animal is said to have been passively immunized. In other words, it has acquired its immunity by merely receiving immune serum from another animal; its part in the procedure has, thus, been a passive one. Treatment of human subjects with diphtheria antitoxin obtained from horses previously immunized with diphtheria toxin is an example of passive immunization. Active immunity, on the other hand, results from the original injections of the antigen. Thus horses inoculated with diphtheria toxin become actively immune to the toxin since they produce their own antitoxin rather than receiving it passively from some other source. While immunity conferred passively is only transient, active immunity is more prolonged. To immunize human subjects actively, and thus more permanently, to diphtheria toxin was the practical objective which Behring was seeking to achieve.

"In a former publication," wrote Theobald Smith in 1909, "I briefly called attention to the fact that an active immunity may be induced in guinea pigs by mixtures of diphtheria toxin and antitoxin which, after subcutaneous injection, produce no local lesion recognizable during the life of the animal, no general disturbances indicated by loss of weight and no paralysis. This acquired immunity lasts at least two years. This phenomenon is of both theoretical and practical importance. As the facts will show, it does not harmonize fully with current theories of the relation between toxins and antitoxins in mixtures. From the practical standpoint, it offers a promising field for investigations in the active immunization of the human subject. If the latter reacts as does the guinea pig, it should be an easy matter to confer a relatively high degree of active immunity lasting several years without any appreciable disturbances of health."

Four years later, in 1913, Behring reported the successful use of toxin-antitoxin mixtures in the immunization of children against diphtheria.[25] During the same year a practical method was discovered for distinguishing non-immune individuals from those already immune to the disease.[26]

Known as the Schick test, it consisted of injecting into the skin a small dose of diphtheria toxin and observing the local reaction. In those whose blood serum contained no antitoxin, a characteristic reddish swelling developed at the site of injection. In those who were immune, the antitoxin already present in the circulation neutralized the injected toxin and prevented the reaction from occurring. By means of this simple test, it was possible to identify the individuals who needed to be immunized.

Although widely used for about a decade, the toxin-antitoxin vaccine was eventually replaced by a chemically modified toxin, known as *toxoid*.[27] This formalin-treated product turned out to be an even safer immunizing antigen and is the one that is used today.

The effectiveness of vaccination against diphtheria was nowhere more convincingly demonstrated than in New York.[28] The practice of immunizing Schick-positive, or non-immune, children was begun in the early 1920s under the leadership of William H. Park. By 1928 half of the children in the city had been inoculated. The effect on the death rate from diphtheria was dramatic. As the proportion of children immunized increased still further, the mortality from the disease decreased almost to the vanishing point. Wherever diphtheria vaccination was vigorously pursued, the same thing happened. Today the disease is prevalent only in those parts of the world where immunization is the exception rather than the rule. In most of the major cities of the United States and western Europe, this once dreaded scourge has been virtually eliminated.

During the long and tedious studies which led to the

triumph of vaccination, two additional facts emerged. The
first had to do with healthy diphtheria carriers, whose

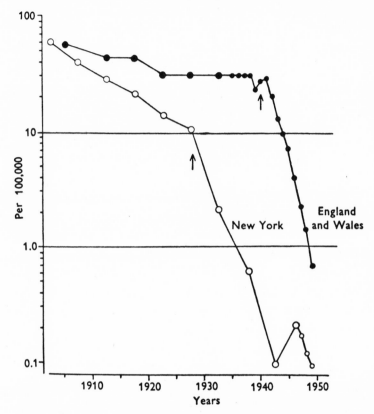

*Figure 11. The death rates per 100,000 from diphtheria in
New York and in England and Wales are plotted on a loga-
rithmic scale for the period 1900–1950. Arrows mark the
years when immunization of 50 percent or more of the children had been reached*

(Reprinted from F. M. Burnett, *Natural History of Infectious
Disease*, Cambridge University Press, 1959.)

existence Löffler had discovered in 1884. Individual throat cultures taken from apparently healthy children revealed that 2 to 5 percent of them carried virulent diphtheria bacilli. The carrier state, however, was eventually found to be relatively transient, usually lasting only two to three weeks. When the throats of all the children in a school, for example, were repeatedly cultured over long periods of time, it was found that the bacilli were passed from one individual to another, so that in the course of a year practically every child in the group had been a carrier.[29] No wonder that diphtheria epidemics spread like wildfire among non-immune children. No wonder that the disease wiped out whole families in the terrible epidemic of 1735. The reason that the families of the ministers who cared for the dying patients were so hard hit is now apparent: as innocent carriers the toiling clergymen often brought home to their own children the virulent bacilli which were killing their patients.

The second fact disclosed during the vaccination studies also concerned epidemiology. In the late 1920s diphtheria in northern England appeared to be considerably more severe than it had been for the previous twenty to thirty years. Despite intensive treatment with antitoxin, a distressing number of children died. A group of bacteriologists at Leeds undertook a detailed study of the diphtheria bacilli which were causing these particularly severe cases and found that they differed from the common form of organism usually found in milder cases.[30] For one thing, the two varieties of bacilli formed different kinds of colonies on solid culture media and thus could be easily recognized. The type associated with the severe cases was given the name *gravis*, while its more benign relative was called *mitis*. Strains of intermediate virulence were described somewhat later and were termed *intermedius*. The discovery of these different types, which are now known to

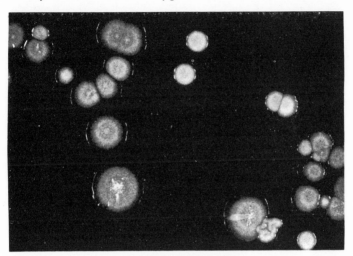

Figure 12. Large and small colonies of diphtheria bacilli on solid culture medium. Gravis and mitis strains exhibit this kind of morphologic difference

(Reprinted from L. Barksdale *et al.*, "Virulence, Toxinogeny, and Lysogeny in *Corynebacterium Diphtheriae*," *Annals of the New York Academy of Sciences*, Vol. LXXXVIII [1960], Art. 5, p. 1093.)

be derived from one another by genetic mutation, created great interest among bacteriologists, since it had always been assumed that all toxin-bearing diphtheria bacilli were the same. Subsequent studies relating to their occurrence have revealed that serious outbreaks of diphtheria, causing a high mortality, are consistently due to either the *gravis* or the *intermedius* types, whereas milder epidemics are usually due to *mitis* strains.[31, 32] Surely the murderous epidemic in Kingston, New Hampshire, must have been caused by *gravis* bacilli!

All that I have related was unknown when the terrible epidemic of throat distemper erupted in the American Colonies in 1735. The utter helplessness of the doctors of the day is poignantly described in the following verses: [33]

> The Doctor's Art, can find no part,
>   nor Cure for this Distemper;
> By Physick long, nor Cordial strong,
>   They cannot find the Center.
>
> It is unknown to any one
>   and all the Doctors skill,
> To cure this Plague, or to engage
>   To cure it at their will.
>
> They're in the dark, in every part,
>   and cannot find it out,
> From where it strikes, and where it lights
>   They cannot point it out.
>
> If we should call the Doctors all
>   and let them all engage,
> We cannot find in any kind
>   That they can cure this Plague.

Now, after only a little more than two hundred years, physicians have at their command all of the scientific facts needed to eradicate diphtheria. Indeed, it has already become a clinical rarity in those areas of the world where modern knowledge has been effectively applied. But the story does not end here, for many questions about mechanisms remain unanswered. The current frontiers of diphtheria research deal more with molecules than with microbes.

MOLECULES

Twenty-five years from now we shall probably know the complete structures of one hundred protein molecules and a few nucleic acid molecules. We shall then have a detailed understanding of the ways in which a few enzymes carry out their specific activities, the way in which genes duplicate themselves and accomplish their individual tasks of precisely controlling the synthesis of protein molecules with well defined structures, the way in which abnormal molecules give rise to the manifestations of the diseases that they cause, the ways in which drugs and other physiologically active substances achieve their effects. When this time comes, medicine will have made a significant start in its transformation from macroscopic and cellular medicine to molecular medicine.

LINUS PAULING (1959)

ONE OF THE MOST constant characteristics of scientific research is its endlessness. Facts learned from experimentation are never ultimate. They always raise new questions, and these, in turn, must be answered by new experiments. The progress of science has been likened to the assembling of a giant jigsaw puzzle, in which the incorporation of each new piece is dependent upon the pieces already in place. As each addition is made, a little more of the total picture emerges. Certain critical insertions complete whole figures or scenes in the growing panorama; others reveal the existence of new vistas, often totally unexpected. Such key pieces, when added to the science puzzle, are usually hailed as great discoveries, but they are not necessarily any greater than the rest. More often than not, their distinction is due to their timeliness.

The story of diphtheria admirably fits this analogy. Behring's first successful vaccine stemmed directly from Theobald Smith's studies of toxin-antitoxin mixtures in America. Smith's work, on the other hand, was dependent upon the discovery of diphtheria toxin by Roux and Yersin at the Pasteur Institute and upon the subsequent production of antitoxin in Germany by Behring and Kitasato. Both of these advances were made feasible by the classic studies of Löffler on the pathogenesis of experimental diphtheria, which, in turn, followed the first description of the diphtheria bacillus by Krebs. In fact, each advance since the time of Hippocrates can readily be shown to have come about only because of some previous discovery. One after another, the individual pieces of the puzzle have gradually been fitted together, so that today we have a relatively clear picture of the whole disease.

Indeed, few human ailments are as well understood as diphtheria. Not only do we know its cause, its mode of transmission, and its mechanism of pathogenesis, but we also have at our disposal effective methods of treating it and preventing it. Despite this impressive body of knowledge, the end is nowhere near in sight, for many problems remain unsolved. It is these problems which concern the modern microbiologist. Just what are some of them and why have they escaped solution?

To answer the second half of the query first, we need only turn to the jigsaw puzzle. Let us examine the edge where the picture of contemporary microbiology seems to be emerging, and where pieces are now falling into place with unusual rapidity. We will notice that the individual pieces are quite different from those put into place by Leeuwenhoek, Löffler, Pasteur, and Koch. The general scene portrayed has far more exquisite detail than is found in the older sections. The units involved are not body cells or microbes in the gross, or poorly defined toxins, or humoral antibodies; instead they are specific molecules, some belonging to the parasite, some to the host, some relatively large, others extremely small, some having to do with pathogenicity, others with immunity, and still others with heredity. If we move along the puzzle's border to the section where microbiology merges with biology, we will find that the same kind of change has taken place. Like modern biology in general, microbiology has "gone molecular." Accordingly, the questions being asked about diphtheria in the 1960s have to do with specific molecules rather than with whole bacterial or host cells. Many of them have not yet been answered because the necessary surrounding pieces, which in many instances have to do with the biochemistry of normal cells, have not yet been put into place at the border of the puzzle. When these have been inserted, answers are sure to follow.

What, then, are the specific questions about diphtheria which modern microbiologists are attempting to answer? Three which seem at the moment to be of particular importance are:

(1) *What makes one strain of diphtheria bacillus produce toxin and another not? In other words, how does the cellular chemistry of a toxin-producing bacillus differ from that of its non-toxigenic relatives?*

(2) *What biochemical factors of the tissue environment influence the amount of toxin produced by each bacillus, and how do they control its rate of synthesis?*

(3) *How do the large protein molecules of the toxin damage the tissue cells, or, to put it more specifically, what is the precise "biochemical lesion" which they initiate?*

It will be noted that all three questions concern diphtheria *toxin*. This is not surprising since the toxin alone may cause the death of the patient. Tragic proof of this fact was provided by an accident which occurred in Japan in 1946.[1] Of four lots of diphtheria toxin being made into toxoid by treatment with formalin, one was inadvertently left untreated. The lot which contained active toxin instead of the less injurious toxoid was used to immunize a large number of children in the Kansai district. Seven hundred became ill and sixty-two died. Any doubt that the purified toxin is lethal for human subjects was dispelled forever.

Let us begin with question number one: what causes a given strain of diphtheria bacillus to produce toxin? The answer, up to a point, is already known and is relatively simple, although admittedly somewhat surprising. In 1951, V. J. Freeman at the University of Washington, in Seattle, made the remarkable discovery that toxigenic diphtheria bacilli are infected by a specific bacterial virus.[2] Later studies by Neal Groman at the same institution have revealed that the virus-toxin relationship is an absolute one.[3] That is, strains which harbor the virus produce toxin, and those free of the virus do not produce toxin. Furthermore, non-toxigenic strains can be made toxigenic by being infected with the virus, and, conversely, toxigenic strains can be rendered non-toxigenic by being freed of the virus.

To explain this remarkable phenomenon more fully, it will be necessary to consider how bacterial viruses behave in their microbial hosts.[4] Like other viruses, they are capable of multiplying only in actively metabolizing cells. To put it another way, they are unable by themselves to synthesize all of the complicated chemical compounds which make up their own structure. Accordingly, they can multiply only by stealing the necessary missing compounds from the "chemical plants" of the cells they invade. As applied to virulent bacterial viruses, the term "steal" is really not strong enough, for what happens is that the virus takes over the microbe's chemical plant and forces it somehow to make virus "building blocks" instead of the compounds needed for its own nutrition. Thus, the virus thrives at the expense of the microbe and literally "eats it out of house and home." When the number of intracellular virus particles has reached a given point, the microbe disintegrates. Because of its bacteriolytic action, a bacterial virus is called a *bacteriophage*, or "eater of bacteria." In scientific language, the term *phage* is used as a convenient abbreviation.

During the past decade a vast body of knowledge has accumulated concerning bacteriophages, primarily because they have turned out to be extraordinarily convenient

organisms to study in the laboratory. Whereas animal
viruses can be grown only in living animals or in relatively
complicated tissue cultures, the phages thrive in simple

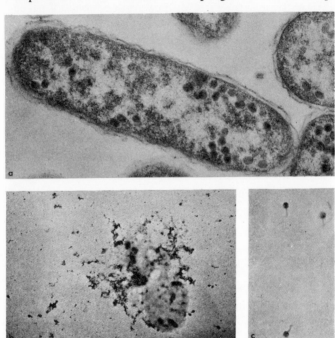

*Figure 13. a. Intracellular growth of phage particles in in-
fected bacillus. b. Bacteriophage causing disintegration of
bacillus. Individual phage particles which have been released
from the cell may be seen scattered through the field.
c. Higher magnification of released phage particles*

(Photograph a. taken by Kellenberger and reprinted from
W. Burrows, *Textbook of Microbiology*, Philadelphia, W. B.
Saunders Company, 1959. Photographs b. and c. taken by S. E.
Luria and T. F. Anderson and reprinted from The Merck
Report, January, 1945.)

broth cultures of bacteria. Thus, bacteriophage technology is surprisingly simple. At the moment, no other living organisms, big or little, are being studied more intensively than bacteriophages. As one investigator has put it, "nothing brings us so close to the riddle of Life—and to its solution —as viruses." [5]

To the microbiologist, phages provide readily manipulated models for studying the mechanisms of viral infection and synthesis. For the geneticist, they make possible the analysis of hereditary phenomena in a matter of hours; if attempted in higher animals, such analyses would require years, decades, or even centuries to complete. In biochemistry and biophysics, they offer an unparalleled opportunity for the study of the complex nucleic acid molecules, known as DNA, which constitute the active genetic material and control critical chemical reactions of living cells, particularly the synthesis of highly specific proteins. And, finally, in cancer research, they have suggested valuable new leads relating to the increasingly attractive hypothesis that many malignancies may be due to so-called "tumor-viruses." Surely, if bacteriophages are so important in contemporary science and, in addition, hold the answer to our question about toxin-production by diphtheria bacilli, we had better pause long enough to take a good look at them.

Although different bacteriophages vary in morphology and do not resemble in structure the more common animal viruses, they are readily seen with the electron microscope. The species which has been most exhaustively studied is one known as T2. This phage, which thrives on a certain

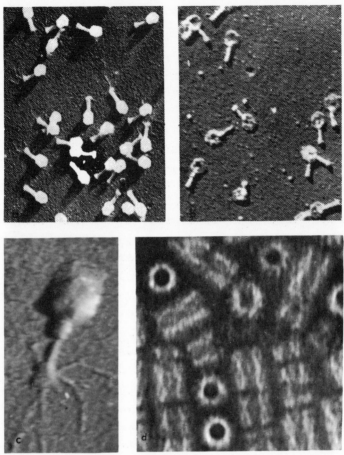

Figure 14. a. Electron photomicrograph of bacteriophage T2. b. "Ghosts" of T2 prepared by osmotic shock which causes phage to discharge the nucleic acid from its polyhedral head. c. Enlarged electron photomicrograph of T2 phage disrupted by treatment with N-ethyl maleimide. d. Purified tail sheaths of T2 phage, some on end showing hollow bore of tail and some lying flat

(a, b. Reprinted from R. M. Herriott and J. L. Barlow, "The

strain of a common intestinal bacterium, has a tadpole-like structure with a polyhedral head, and a short rod-shaped tail at the end of which may be seen a number of thin filaments. When infecting a bacterial cell, the T2 phage first becomes attached by the tip of its tail to the bacterial surface. A few minutes later the DNA contained in its polyhedral head is discharged into the bacterial cytoplasm, leaving behind, on the surface of the bacterium, the outer protein coat of the phage particle. As if by a syringe and needle, the phage DNA is thus injected into the bacterial cell. The tail through which the DNA passes can be seen to be a hollow tube. Its distal end is thought to contain a tiny plug, which is somehow released during the act of injection.

After the reproductively essential DNA of the phage has entered the bacterial cell, there follows a latent period of about twenty minutes, during which time no new infective phage particles appear in the culture. Meanwhile, however, a number of important things happen to the bacterial host cell. First, it promptly ceases to divide. Second, it stops making its own DNA and starts synthesizing phage DNA and phage protein. Third, after ap-

―――――

Protein Coats of 'Ghosts' of Coliphage T2. I. Preparation, Assay and Some Chemical Properties," *Journal of General Physiology*, Vol. XL [1957], No. 5, pp. 809–825.

c. Reprinted with permission from C. B. Anfinsen, *The Molecular Basis of Evolution*, New York, John Wiley & Sons, Inc., 1959.

d. Reprinted from S. Brenner *et al.*, "Structural Components of Bacteriophage," *Journal of Molecular Biology*, I [1959], 281.)

proximately ten minutes, complete phage particles begin
to appear in its cytoplasm, where they multiply rapidly.
And, finally, when their number has reached about a

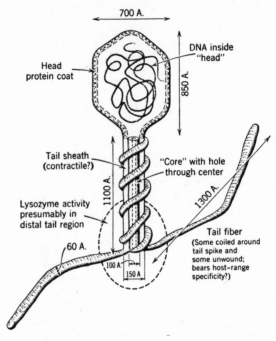

*Figure 15. Diagram of T2 bacteriophage. A. refers to Ang-
ströms which are units of linear measurement equivalent to
one hundred-millionth of a centimeter*

(Reprinted with permission from C. B. Anfinsen, *The Molecular Basis of Evolution,* New York, John Wiley & Sons, Inc.,
1959.)

hundred, the bacterial cell disintegrates, and the newly
formed phage particles are released into the surrounding
medium.

All of this will take place only in an actively growing culture of bacteria. If the metabolism of the bacterial cell is sufficiently interfered with by some outside agent, such

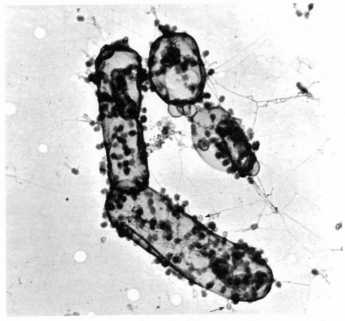

Figure 16. Electron photomicrograph of T2 bacteriophage adsorbed onto surface of colon bacilli. Some of the adsorbed phage particles (see arrows) have already discharged their DNA into the bacterial cell

(Reprinted with permission from C. B. Anfinsen, *The Molecular Basis of Evolution*, New York, John Wiley & Sons, Inc., 1959.)

as an antibiotic, the bacteria stop multiplying, and the production of bacteriophage also ceases. Thus, it is clear that the phage particles are not capable of multiplying

by themselves, but are literally made by the bacteria. It
is equally evident that the factor which causes the bacterial
cell to make bacteriophage at the expense of its own multi-

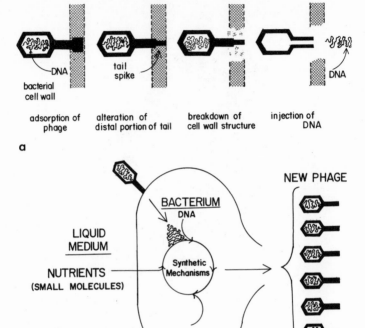

*Figure 17. a. Diagram of manner in which phage discharges
its DNA into bacterial cell. b. Schematic diagram of metabolic action of phage DNA on infected bacterial cell*

plication is the DNA injected from the head of the original
phage.

Once the virulent phage particles of the type described
are released into the medium, they infect new bacterial

cells and thus eventually bring about the destruction of all the bacteria in the culture. When the bacteria are cultured on a solid medium rather than in liquid broth, only those in the immediate vicinity of each phage particle are disintegrated, or *lysed*. The resulting clear areas, in

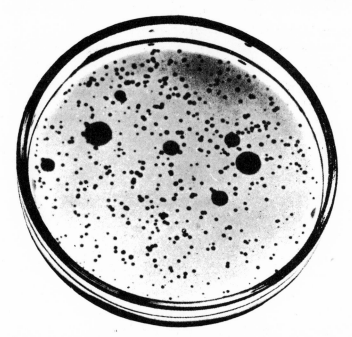

Figure 18. Bacterial "lawn" infected with bacteriophage growing on solid nutrient medium in glass Petri dish. The small holes, or plaques, in the confluent lawn of colon bacilli have been produced by T2 bacteriophage; the larger plaques are due to a related phage strain known as T3

(Reprinted from W. Weidel, *Virus*, Ann Arbor, University of Michigan Press, 1959, by permission of Springer-Verlag, Heidelberg.)

the otherwise continuous sheet of bacteria growing on the surface of the solid medium, are known as plaques. Since each bacteria-free plaque is caused by a single phage particle, the number of plaques on the plate indicates the number of phage particles in the bacterial suspension originally placed on the plate. Thus individual phage particles can be counted and quantitation becomes relatively simple.

Some species of bacteriophage, however, are not virulent; that is, they do not cause lysis of the bacteria which they invade. These avirulent species are capable of setting up housekeeping in a bacterial cell without harming it. Although they infect the cell by the same "syringe and needle" mechanism as do their virulent cousins, their DNA behaves quite differently inside the bacterial cell. Instead of "taking over" the chemical plant and forcing it to make bacteriophage particles to the exclusion of bacterial foodstuffs, the phage DNA becomes incorporated into the genetic apparatus of the cell. There, as an integral part of the bacterial chromosome, it is passed on to each generation of daughter cells without interfering with multiplication. If such a daughter cell is sufficiently harmed by unfavorable cultural conditions, the dormant phage DNA molecule will become reactivated and will force the cell to produce virulent bacteriophage particles which will eventually cause it to lyse. Because bacterial cells which harbor the masked bacteriophage virus retain this lytic potentiality, the cells are said to be *lysogenic*, and the phenomenon, as a whole, is called *lysogeny*.

But how does lysogeny relate to the virulence of diphtheria bacilli? The answer lies in a second phenomenon known as *lysogenic conversion*.[6] When a bacterial cell is infected with an avirulent bacteriophage, it not only becomes lysogenic, but it also may acquire the capability of synthesizing one or more chemical constituents which it is unable to make in the absence of the virus. In other words, the incorporation of the phage DNA into its genetic apparatus so alters the cell's metabolic machinery as to cause it to produce a new metabolite. In the case of lysogenic diphtheria bacilli which are infected by a specific avirulent bacteriophage known as the β *phage*, the new metabolite formed is the all-important disease-producing

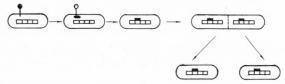

Figure 19. Schematic representation of lysogeny, showing relationship of phage DNA to chromosomal apparatus of bacterial cell

toxin. Thus, the virulence of the organism is directly dependent upon the presence of the β phage in its chromosomes. If, for any reason, the β phage is eliminated, the organism ceases to produce toxin and thereby loses its virulence. In a sense, then, only diphtheria bacilli which harbor a masked virus infection of their own are capable of causing diphtheria.

Strange as this relationship may seem, it is quite in keeping with current concepts of cellular chemistry. Diphtheria toxin is nothing more than a highly complex specific protein molecule synthesized by the diphtheria bacillus;[7] and, there is abundant evidence that the synthesis of cellular proteins is somehow controlled by the nucleic acid or DNA content of the chromosomes.[8] Accordingly, it is not surprising that the incorporation of β phage DNA into the chromosomal apparatus of a previously non-toxic strain of diphtheria bacillus should render it capable of producing the noxious toxin. Just how the specific structures of the chromosomal DNA molecules control the synthesis of each of the myriads of individual proteins formed by metabolizing cells is not yet known. But the evidence that they do exert such a control is most convincing.

The practical importance of this fascinating phenomenon is illustrated by the following case history recorded during World War I.[9] At the Royal Naval College in Greenwich, a Surgeon Commander, Sir Sheldon F. Dudley, made an exhaustive study of diphtheria carriers among recruits. On frequent occasions he isolated diphtheria bacilli from the throats of apparently healthy trainees. Some of the strains which he cultured were found to produce toxin; others were non-toxigenic and thus avirulent. On every occasion in which a virulent or toxigenic organism was isolated, the individual involved was found to be immune—that is, his blood serum contained appreciable amounts of antitoxin, which protected him against the disease. Many of the recruits who harbored avirulent organisms, on the other hand, were non-immune. These results seemed altogether logical. Then something totally unexpected happened. One of the non-immune individuals, who had been carrying an avirulent bacillus in his throat for more than two months, suddenly came down with diphtheria. When his throat was recultured, he was found to be infected with a toxin-

producing strain which, except for its toxigenicity, appeared
to be identical with the original avirulent one. What had
happened to this organism to make it suddenly produce
toxin? At the time, no explanation could be given, but
today the answer appears to be obvious. Either the carrier
strain itself became infected with the β phage, or else the
patient became newly infected with a phage-bearing strain
which was otherwise indistinguishable from the original
strain. In either event, the presence in his throat of diphtheria bacilli superinfected with the β virus promptly caused
the patient to come down with the disease.

Let us now turn to the second question relating to diphtheria toxin, which concerns the influence of chemical
environment upon its production. The key factor here
appears to be the chemical element iron. Its importance
was first suggested in a surprisingly roundabout way.[10]
As soon as diphtheria toxoid had been shown to be an
effective immunizing agent, pharmaceutical companies
undertook to produce it commerically. At the start, little
was known about the chemistry of the process, except
that the growing bacilli needed a nutritious culture medium
and an abundant supply of oxygen. The bacteriologists of
the Connaught firm, in Toronto, developed a highly
successful growth medium containing self-digested pig
stomachs. The toxin yields with this medium were the
highest ever reported. When laboratories in other cities
tried to adopt the Connaught method, however, they were
unable to produce a potent toxin. Clearly, there was something missing in their cultures, and this something seemed

to be peculiar to Toronto. Eventually the difficulty was traced to the water used in the culture media. Toronto tap water was exceptionally "hard" and contained a high concentration of calcium, which reacted with the phosphate from the pig stomach digest to form a precipitate. The calcium phosphate precipitate, in turn, carried down most of the iron from the medium and rendered it satisfactory for toxin production.

This important relationship between iron and toxin production has since been exhaustively studied by Alwin Pappenheimer.[11] Inasmuch as living cells possess iron-containing catalysts essential for respiration, they naturally require traces of iron for growth. The diphtheria bacillus is no exception. In a culture medium completely free of iron, the organism fails to grow. When the iron content of the medium is gradually increased from zero to one part per ten million, the bacterial growth improves. Concomitantly, as might be expected, there is an increase in toxin production. At iron concentrations above this level, however, the bacterial growth continues to increase, but the formation of toxin begins to decline. When the concentration of iron has reached six parts per ten million, the yield of toxin becomes negligible. Somehow the presence of too much iron in the medium causes the growing organisms to desist from making their lethal poison. Indeed, it has been shown that each individual bacillus makes toxin only when the iron supply in its environment has become practically exhausted, and its own intracellular iron has fallen to a very low level. Thus, it is possible to attain maximum toxin production in the laboratory only when the iron content of the culture medium is limited to precisely the right amount.

The results of Pappenheimer's systematic studies have greatly facilitated the commercial production of diphtheria toxoid. At the same time, they have posed a baffling question

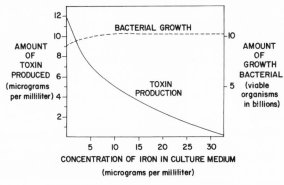

Figure 20. Relation of iron content of culture medium to growth and toxin production of diphtheria bacillus

(Data plotted from M. Yoneda and A. M. Pappenheimer, Jr., "Some Effects of Iron Deficiency on the Extracellular Products Released by Toxigenic and Non-toxigenic Strains of *Corynebacterium Diphtheriae*," *Journal of Bacteriology*, LXXIV [1957], 256.)

to clinicians and pathologists. How, it may be asked, do diphtheria bacilli manage to produce toxin in the throats of patients where the iron content of the tissues is well above the level which depresses the formation of toxin in the test tube? At present it is possible only to offer a speculative answer. The most logical explanation appears to lie in the nature of the relatively thick diphtheritic membrane which forms on the surface of the infected tissues. This membrane is devoid of a blood supply and is composed primarily of fibrin and dead or dying cells. Its nature suggests that it may be relatively impermeable to the diffusion of hemoglobin and other iron-containing substances from the viable tissues upon which it is deposited. Since the diphtheria bacilli can be seen under the microscope to be concentrated on the outer surface of the membrane (Fig. 10), it may be postulated that the supply of iron available to them may readily become exhausted and thus permit the production of toxin.[6] Whether this explanation is correct remains to be proved.

We come now to the last and most complicated of the three questions about diphtheria toxin: how does it injure tissue cells?

The two most striking properties of diphtheria toxin are its extreme potency and the relative slowness with which it acts. Less than one ten-thousandth of a gram of the toxin injected beneath the skin will kill a 250-gram guinea pig.[6] It has been calculated that the number of molecules that will cause irreparable damage to an individual guinea pig cell is probably less than ten.[12] Not all animals, however, are equally susceptible to the toxin. Mouse cells, for example, are more than a thousand times as resistant as the cells of guinea pigs. Man, unfortunately, reacts more like the guinea pig than the mouse. It can be calculated from the Kansai tragedy, referred to earlier, that an ounce of the toxin would be more than enough to kill everyone in the city of New York. Clearly, both the extraordinary degree of toxicity and the remarkable variance of species susceptibility must be accounted for by the manner in which the toxin acts. As to the slowness of its action, investigators have long known that a latent period of five to six hours always elapses before guinea pigs given thousands of lethal doses manifest the first signs of illness.[6] Similarly, toxin-treated cells taken from even the most susceptible animal show no visible signs of damage for as long as four or five hours.[13] What goes on during this relatively prolonged latent period? Obviously, critical biochemical events which are intimately involved in the toxin's mode of action must be in progress. It is these molecular events which concern the modern students of diphtheria.

One of the first leads as to what may transpire in the latent period came from Pappenheimer's work on the iron problem. In culture filtrates which contained large amounts of toxin previous investigators had noted the presence of a pinkish pigment known as *coproporphyrin*.[14] Since coproporphyrin is a chemical precursor of an important group of cellular respiratory enzymes called *cytochromes*, Pappenheimer reasoned that diphtheria toxin might be chemically related to a part of the cytochrome molecule. This thought was substantiated by the fact that cytochrome molecules are composed of two distinct constituents: one, an iron-containing pigment closely related to coproporphyrin; the other, a protein of the general nature of diphtheria toxin. Furthermore, he noted that the more toxin and coproporphyrin a given diphtheria bacillus produced, the less cytochrome it contained within its own cytoplasm. Thus, it appeared that when the organism was grown in the absence of an excess of iron, it stopped making its own cytochrome and produced, instead, coproporphyrin and

diphtheria toxin. From these findings Pappenheimer concluded that diphtheria toxin may be so similar in chemical
structure to the protein portion of the cytochrome enzymes
that it is able to block their vital action in other animal
cells.[15]

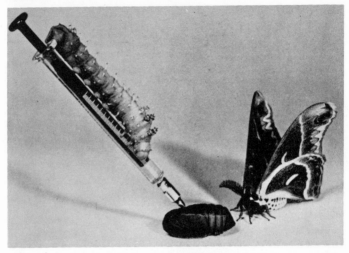

*Figure 21. Cecropia silkworm used by Pappenheimer to study
effect of diphtheria toxin on cytochrome system. The three
stages of its life cycle are indicated by: the caterpillar on the
syringe at the left; the pupa, which is being injected below;
and the adult moth on the right*

(Reprinted from A. M. Pappenheimer, Jr., "The Diphtheria
Toxin," *Scientific American*, October, 1952, p. 32.)

To test this interesting hypothesis, he turned to the
study of a most unusual laboratory animal—the cecropia
silkworm.[16] As every biologist knows, this insect goes
through three stages in its life history—from caterpillar,
to pupa, to moth. Striking biochemical changes occur in

the tissues during the various stages of the metamorphosis. The abundant caterpillar musculature, which is rich in cytochrome, disappears at the time of pupation. In the dormant pupa, what little cytochrome remains is concentrated in a small group of muscles in the abdomen. As adult development begins, there is a resurgence of cytochrome formation which persists until the adult moth is fully formed. Pappenheimer's experiments with *Cecropia* consisted of testing the resistance of the insect to diphtheria toxin at each of its three stages of metamorphosis. The differences noted were striking. In the dormant pupal stage, when the tissues were relatively devoid of cytochrome, the resistance to the toxin was a hundred to a thousand times greater than in either of the high cytochrome stages. Furthermore, in the injected pupae, the only tissues affected by the toxin were the cytochrome-containing abdominal muscles. Not only did they become paralyzed when the pupa was injected with toxin, but they eventually disintegrated in marked contrast to the cytochrome-free heart muscle, which remained apparently unaffected.

The results of these ingenious experiments strongly suggest that diphtheria toxin does indeed exert a profound effect upon the normal functioning of the cytochrome system of enzymes. Just where this action takes place in the animal cell and how it influences metabolic reactions upon which the vitality of the cell depends has been discovered only within the past few months. Three new observations have just been published. All three have been made on isolated cells grown in tissue culture. They may be briefly summarized as follows:

First, it has been shown by Norman Strauss and Edelmira Hendee that toxin-treated cells stop synthesizing protein several hours before they begin to exhibit any morphological signs of damage under the microscope.[13] Since protein molecules are among the most important building

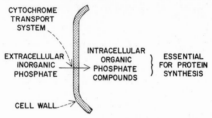

Figure 22. Schematic diagram of role of cytochrome in transporting inorganic phosphorus across cell wall. Latest evidence suggests that diphtheria toxin damages cell by blocking action of cytochrome transport system at surface of wall, thus depriving the cell of phosphorus compounds needed for synthesis of proteins and other essential constituents

blocks of all living cells, it follows that such an inhibition of protein synthesis must eventually be lethal.

Second, Strauss and Hendee have demonstrated that during the first hour of its action the deleterious effect of the toxin can be reversed by antitoxin.[13] The manner in which this reversal takes place strongly suggests that the toxin acts at the surface of the cell rather than at some locus within its cytoplasm.

Third, Iwao Kato and Alwin Pappenheimer have found that the primary effect of the toxin, which takes place almost immediately, is not upon protein synthesis *per se*, but rather upon the cellular incorporation of inorganic phosphate molecules, which, in turn, are needed for the process of making the protein.[17] Since cytochrome enzymes are involved in the active transport of inorganic phosphate across the cell membrane, it is now postulated that diphtheria toxin exerts its damaging effect by inhibiting the action of cytochrome at the cell surface, thus breaking a vital chain of biochemical reactions necessary for the formation of essential intracellular components, including proteins. That the theory may indeed be valid is further suggested by the observation that cells taken from a toxin-resistant animal, such as the mouse, continue to assimilate inorganic phosphate and form new protein, even in the presence of large amounts of toxin. This finding, which in a sense is the most interesting of all, is in keeping with the notoriously variable effect of diphtheria toxin on animals of different species.

So the knowledge of diphtheria has progressed from miasmas to molecules. The resulting practical benefits to mankind have been immense. But the story of diphtheria is only one example of the progress of medical science. The acquisition of new knowledge in all of the branches of medicine has revolutionized the treatment and prevention of disease. From this very revolution, however, have come new problems to the medical profession—problems which are primarily social rather than scientific.

CONSEQUENCES

For everything you gain, you lose something.
RALPH WALDO EMERSON

LATE IN 1960 the editors of *Harper's Magazine* published a special supplement entitled "The Crisis in American Medicine." [1] In introducing it to their readers, they made two statements: first, that "American medicine is the best in the world"; and, second, that millions of Americans are "bitterly dissatisfied with the medical care they are getting." Despite its unbecoming immodesty, the first of these assertions may conceivably be correct, although, as I shall point out, it is open to challenge, particularly in Scandinavia. What is not debatable is the fact that world medicine is better today than ever before, because of the kinds of scientific advance illustrated by the story of diphtheria. Therefore, the second statement comes as a shock. Why should Americans be dissatisfied with their medical care? The answers lie in a whole series of new problems created by the very progress that has advanced medicine.

The most important of these troublesome developments are:

(1) The changing relationship of the physician to his patients

(2) An impending shortage of doctors

(3) The rising costs of medical care

(4) The "two-culture" trend within the profession

You will note that I have omitted two other topics of great importance—those of birth control and death control, or euthanasia. The former is now being widely discussed, particularly in relation to population pressures. I shall not consider it here because many factors other than advances in medicine are responsible for the current "population explosion." The increasing need for an acceptable system of euthanasia, on the other hand, is directly related to the capability of the modern doctor to control so many acute illnesses and thus, as one perceptive writer has put it, to "prolong the deaths" of so many patients.[1] I have chosen not to include it because the issue involved is essentially a moral one, and is not likely to be resolved until the problems created by unwanted survival become considerably more pressing than they are today.

First, to comprehend the change which has taken place in the doctor-patient relationship, one need only examine the primary role of the physician of the last century. Imagine, for a moment, what it must have been like for the doctor of 1890 to be called to the bedside of a child with laryngeal diphtheria. How much could he do for the patient? If well trained, he would recognize the signs and symptoms of the disease and thus make the correct diagnosis. But then what? Knowing the contagiousness of diphtheria, he would explain to the worried parents the danger of cross-infection and would warn them against allowing the other children to enter the sickroom. He would instruct the mother about washing her hands after caring for the patient. He would show her how to apply cool compresses to the child's forehead to allay the fever. If the cough was distressing or restlessness became severe, he might prescribe a sedative. But as for influencing the progress of the disease itself, he would be virtually helpless. He would have no injectable antiserum with which to combat the devastating toxin in the patient's bloodstream. Without antimicrobial drugs, he would have no way of stopping the growth of the diphtheria bacilli in the throat. In short, he could only wait and hope.

If the fates were kind, the child would slowly recover, perhaps completely or perhaps with some residual paralysis. But if they were unkind, the disease would proceed relentlessly on its course. In the end, death might come suddenly from toxemia, or it might mercifully end a long and losing struggle against obstruction of the airway. Even if suffocation were prevented by a desperate tracheotomy, secondary pneumonia would probably develop, and the outcome would be the same.

Before the long vigil was over, however, the doctor would have made many visits to the bedside, he would have come to know every member of the family, and he would have done all in his power to relieve the dying child. Despite his failure to check the illness, the parents would be everlastingly grateful for his comforting efforts. Later, when beset by some other adversity, whether related to sickness or not, they would turn to him for help. And so it would be with each family he served; in time he would become one of the most beloved figures in his community.

That science has changed all this, there is no doubt. The altered social status of the doctor results, in the words of a contemporary clinician, from "the change in the nature of medical practice from an intensely personal service to the objective and highly intellectualized approach demanded by the sophistication of modern biological theory. Nor can we expect," he continues, "the old unqualified admiration of the layman. He reads the *Reader's Digest* too, and he knows about research. He no longer feels that his health has been salvaged or his life saved by the physician's personal effort alone." [1]

Today's doctor no longer performs as a soloist. To do his job now, he must have the cooperation of other physicians, of nurses, of expert technicians, of hospital orderlies, and of community health officials. In cases of serious illness he usually functions as a member of a team, of which, to be sure, he is still the captain. But his contact with the patient and the family is far less intimate than in the past. Although he can cure many physical ills, he does so through effective drugs or operations rather than through long hours of personal care. His patients come to him far more often than he goes to them. The place of meeting is usually an office or a hospital room rather than the intimate confines of the home. Also, much of his work is preventive and therefore less dramatic. Indeed, there should never be a case of diphtheria among his clientele, for a simple injection or two will prevent it. As his tools have become more effective, the number of patients he can care for has increased. And as the time that he gives to each individual has lessened, so have his services become less intimate.

Naturally, this change has been accepted with great reluctance by the public, for the average person feels that what he has gained in physical well-being he has lost in moral support. Indeed, the doctor of fifty years ago often had little to offer *but* moral support, and this he gave superbly. The primary task of today's physician, however, is very different, and it is different because of the progress of science.

Unfortunately, the change has given rise to a widespread misconception concerning the compatibility of scientific training and human sympathy. One often hears the thoughtless accusation that scientists lack compassion. Such a general incrimination is, of course, absurd. It is made most often by those who feel scientifically insecure. An increasing knowledge of science will no more blunt the sensibilities of an understanding clinician than participation in clinical practice will warm the heart of an unresponsive scientist. What the effective doctor must have today is the combination of a hard head and a soft heart. I recently heard a distinguished physicist put it this way: "Man's astonishing accomplishments in the field of health have come neither from curiosity nor from compassion but rather from a combination of them both."

The second consequence of the scientific revolution in medicine is an impending shortage of doctors. Though not peculiar to the United States, this threat has been given wide publicity in the American press. It stems directly from an ever increasing demand for the vastly improved services which contemporary medicine provides. These services are now looked upon as the inalienable right of every citizen of the nation. Recent statistics indicate that the average American consults a physician five times a year.[2] Education of the general public in matters of hygiene, improved standards of living, the growth of group insurance, and the desire of organized labor for proper medical care have all contributed to the increasing demand for health services. But the most important factor of all has been the success of medical research which has made possible the prevention and cure of so many diseases.

The greater effectiveness of modern medicine has itself served to magnify the problem. For the control of illness has been at least *one* of the factors involved in the current population boom. The life expectancy of Americans, as everyone knows, has risen from forty-seven years in 1900 to over seventy in 1960. Most of this rise has been created by a sharp decline in the death rate of children. In fact, of the twenty-three years gained *in toto*, only four and a half have been added to the lives of persons over forty-five. Most of the change in the child-age group has, in turn, been caused by the control of communicable diseases, including diphtheria. As recently as 1920, American physicians reported 148,000 cases of diphtheria; in 1959 they reported less than a thousand.[2]

Improved medical care has affected the population of the nation in two ways: it has contributed toward the rise in the total census, and it has caused a shift in age distribution, resulting in a higher percentage of the very young and the very old. Since these are the segments of the population that need the most medical attention, it is evident that a double burden has been thrown upon the profession.

How many doctors, then, do we need today? This question is not easy to answer. Two statistical facts are often quoted: first, although the ratio of physicians to patients in this country rose slightly between 1931 and 1940, it has since shown a definite decline; and, second,

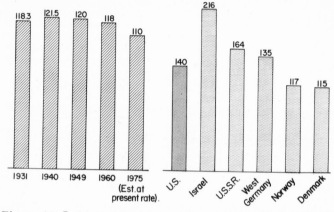

Figure 23. Left: past, present, and projected figures relating to the number of practicing physicians per 100,000 population in the United States excluding retired and Federal employees. Right: comparison of physician-population ratio in United States with those of other countries. Figures represent number of physicians per 100,000 population

(Reprinted from the New York *Times*, November 6, 1960.)

the number of physicians per 100,000 population in both Israel and the Soviet Union is appreciably higher than in the United States.[3] Manifestly, figures of this kind may be grossly misleading. For one thing, they tell us nothing about quality. In addition, they offer no clue as to whether the increased efficiency of modern practice may not more than compensate for the increasing demands of the changing population. How does one explain, for example, the fact that life expectancy at birth in Denmark and Norway is even higher than in the United States, despite their appreciably lower ratios of doctors to patients? [2] Is this not an indication that we might improve the utilization of our own physicians?

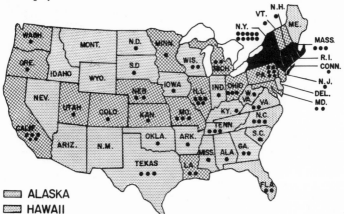

ALASKA
HAWAII

Physicians per 100,000 population
■ Over 150   ▨ 100-149   ▢ Below 100 (U.S. average, 118)
• Medical schools

Figure 24. Map showing distribution of practicing physicians in the various states of the nation

(Reprinted from the New York *Times*, November 6, 1960.)

There is no denying the fact that improper distribution is a major factor in the impending doctor shortage. But even if this defect could somehow be remedied, it is almost certain that the total number of physicians available will soon be too small to meet the nation's needs, for the population is increasing much faster than the number of medical graduates. In 1960, for example, the eighty-odd medical schools of the United States graduated approximately 7,500 students. Judging from the present population trend, we shall have to graduate 11,000 annually by 1975 if we are merely to maintain the present ratio. Projections indicate that we shall meet less than 75 percent of the figure unless we either increase substantially the enrollment of our

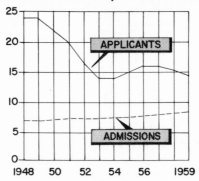

Figure 25. Graph showing decrease in number of applicants to American medical schools. Figures represent number of applicants in thousands

(Reprinted from the New York *Times*, November 6, 1960.)

present schools or create twenty to twenty-five new ones.[4] To do the former would impair the quality of the education offered; to do the latter would cost an estimated billion dollars. Neither course, therefore, looks particularly inviting. A judicious combination of the two will probably be required.

Two additional facets of the doctor-shortage problem are particularly worrisome. The first concerns the decrease in the number of college students who are applying for admission to American medical schools. In 1948 there were 24,000; by 1958 the number had fallen to 15,000.[5] Although this is still twice the number of first-year places available in our medical schools, the trend is a disturbing one, particularly in view of the projected needs for the future. Part of the difficulty is financial, for, unlike doctoral candidates in other branches of science, medical students are not eligible for Federal fellowships. The monetary pressures involved in the training of a doctor are clearly indicated by the fact that 40 percent of all medical students come from families with annual incomes of $10,000 or more,

HEALTH SERVICE

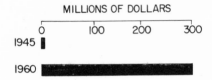

Figure 26. Increase in Public Health Service research expenditures over the past fifteen years

(Data taken from "Final Report of the Study Group on Mission and Organization of the Public Health Service," U.S. Government Printing Office, June 7, 1960, 0-553903.)

whereas only 8 percent of all families in the country have such incomes. Furthermore, a recent survey has shown that 50 percent of our present-day students are in debt at the time of graduation from medical school.[4]

The second facet concerns the tremendous expansion of medical research which has occurred in the United States since World War II. Its growth is indicated by the increasing research budgets of the Public Health Service, since this agency provides more than half of all the dollars now being spent on medical research. In 1945 the Service's research budget totaled about three million dollars; in 1960 it was over three hundred million.[6] Much of the increment in funds is being spent on clinical studies performed in hospitals, under the direction of clinically trained physicians. Because of the time-consuming nature of this investigative work, the physicians involved must inevitably devote less time to clinical practice. The inroad thus made on the nation's pool of practicing physicians is considerable.

When all of these complex factors are weighed, it appears inescapable that we shall soon have a serious shortage of doctors, unless prompt and vigorous action is taken to prevent it. This prospect is highly disturbing to a public accustomed to effective medical care. No wonder there is talk of a *crisis*. And once more let me emphasize that practically all of the causes of this problem are direct consequences of the progress of science.

The third of the difficulties which I listed is so familiar to everyone that I shall do little more than mention it. During the past decade medical costs have increased faster than any other part of the cost-of-living index.[2] Compared to a rise of 26.5 percent in consumer prices since 1947–49, the cost of medical care has risen more than 56 percent. Hospital room rates have increased 120 percent over the same period. Despite the growth of hospital, surgical, and "major medical" insurance, the great bulk of the population is still poorly protected against the catastrophic expense of serious illness. Why have the costs risen so rapidly? The reasons, of course, are many. Some have to do with the general inflationary trend of the past decade, but others are peculiar to medicine itself. And these latter increases have resulted primarily from advances in medical science —advances which have led to new but expensive drugs, new and costly diagnostic, laboratory, and operating room equipment, new and often prolonged methods of hospital therapy, and new but economically burdensome public health programs for the prevention of disease. So here, too, scientific advance is a principal cause of the trouble.

Last, we come to what I have termed the "two-culture" trend within the profession. I refer, of course, to what C. P. Snow has so eloquently defined in his Rede Lecture of 1959, entitled *The Two Cultures and the Scientific Revolution*.[7] This now famous treatise clearly describes the barrier which has arisen between the worlds of science and literature—a barrier in communications resulting primarily from explosive advances in the natural sciences. "The non-scientists," writes Snow, "have a rooted impression that the scientists are shallowly optimistic, unaware of man's condition. On the other hand, the scientists believe that the literary intellectuals are totally lacking in foresight, peculiarly unconcerned with their brother men, in a deep sense anti-intellectual, anxious to restrict both art and thought to the existential moment. . . . Anyone with a mild talent for invective could produce plenty of this kind of subterranean back-chat. On each side there is some of it which is not entirely baseless. It is all destructive. Much of it rests on misrepresentations which are dangerous."

Precisely the same thing has happened within the field of medicine, on a more restricted scale. Here the barrier is between the practicing physician and the medical scientist. How can these two kinds of doctor understand each other's languages when their jobs have become so different? No longer can major discoveries in medicine be made by merely treating patients, for the descriptive phase of medical science has passed. The pressing research problems of the day concern disease mechanisms, which can be studied effectively only with the most precise tools of modern biology, chemistry, physics, and mathematics. But the practicing physician must care for his patients. His approach must be essentially pragmatic. He cannot worry about the fine structure of cellular chromosomes when confronted with a patient suffering from intestinal obstruction. Nor will a knowledge of lysogeny help him to save the life of a child with diphtheria. He must minister to the whole patient. He must treat the mind as well as the body; he must comfort as well as cure. How, then, can he fully appreciate the other culture—the culture of medical science? And yet, as the story of diphtheria has told us, it is precisely this which he must do, if he is to bring to his patients the best that modern medicine has to offer. Whenever he does less, he has failed in his primary mission. Here, then, is the modern doctor's dilemma. What a pity that we have no Bernard Shaw to dramatize this one!

How serious, you may ask, is the two-culture problem in medicine? Is it a real cause for concern? There can be no doubt that it is. In fact, for the doctor it is the most serious of all the consequences of the scientific advance. At the moment, its impact is most keenly felt among medical educators who must find the solution, just as education in general must heal the schism between science and literature.[8]

Naturally enough, opinions are divided as to what should be done to close the gap between practice and research. One school of thought is represented by a Harvard professor, Dr. David Rutstein[1]. He takes the position that the two-culture break among doctors is here to stay. Accepting it as inevitable, he advocates two kinds of curriculum in medical schools—one stressing the practical aspects of medicine, designed for future practitioners; the other emphasizing the basic science background needed by future investigators. At first this suggestion sounds fairly logical, but let us examine it for a moment. What would result if such a course were followed? Obviously, the two-culture split would be further exaggerated. Two kinds of doctor would emerge—one, the healers, trained primarily in the practical clinical methods of the day; the other, the future researchers, schooled in the principles of modern science, some of which, at the moment, have little relevance to the practice of medicine. The question which must be asked here is: how effective would the first of these species be ten years after graduation from medical school? The answer was clearly stated by a member of the Columbia University faculty more than fifteen years ago. In his widely read book *Teacher in America*, Jacques Barzun wrote: "For it is the oldest fallacy about schooling to suppose that it can train a man for 'practical life.' Inevitably while the plan of study is being taught, 'practical life' has moved

on." [9] Certainly, no experienced clinician needs to be re-
minded that what was practical yesterday may be obsolete
tomorrow.[10]

Fortunately for the future of American medicine, there
are physicians who agree with Dean Barzun and take the
position diametrically opposed to that expressed by Dr.
Rutstein. One of the most articulate of these is also a
member of the Columbia faculty, Dr. Dana Atchley. On
frequent occasions his facile pen has inscribed on the pages
of the *Saturday Review*,[11] the *Atlantic Monthly*,[12] and
numerous medical journals the strongest kind of plea for
more science in medicine. And surely his word should carry
weight, for he is one of the nation's most distinguished
practitioners. Far from being an "ivory tower" scientist,
he has devoted his life to the care of patients. The dominant
theme of all of his writings has been that the Healer and
the Scientist can be, and indeed must be, one.

That my own thoughts on this matter are in harmony
with those of Dean Barzun and Dr. Atchley is already
evident. I have stated elsewhere that the greatest advances
in medical practice during the present century have come
not from specific discoveries such as those of anesthesia,
insulin, or modern antimicrobial drugs but rather from
the fact that doctors have been forced by the pressures
of progress to become better scientists.[13] If asked to state
my credo of medicine, I would try to say just that. Only
I should probably ask Dr. Atchley to write the statement
for me.

That the two-culture dilemma of medicine will eventually be met by instilling more science into clinical practice

rather than less, I have not the slightest doubt. In the same way the broader problem of harmonizing the sciences and the humanities must in the end be solved by bringing more humanities to the scientists and more science to the humanists. In fact, the situation is not quite as bleak as portrayed by Professor Snow. There have always been Leonardos and Thomas Jeffersons and Hans Zinssers and C. P. Snows who have easily spanned the gap between the two cultures. And surely there will be many more of them. What is often forgotten is that as knowledge grows, education improves—or at least should improve. For when facts are known, teaching can become more efficient. It does not follow that the study of science stifles interest in the humanities. Indeed, the reverse is usually true. Was the streetcar conductor of yesterday more cultured than the jet pilot of today? Certainly he needed to know much less science; but the fact is, he knew less of everything else, simply because he had not had as good an education. The real questions before us are: How good are we willing to make our system of education? What kind of priority will we give it in terms of time, talent, dollars, and prestige?

And this brings me back to the second and third consequences of the scientific revolution in medicine—the impending shortage of physicians and the rising cost of medical care. They, too, raise questions of priority. If we are willing to provide the funds necessary to construct new medical schools, to enlarge the present ones, and to create enough scholarships for medical students and hospital house officers, there will be no doctor shortage. If we fail to do this, we shall certainly have one. The same principle applies to the cost of medical care. If we are unwilling to pay for the kind of health insurance that will meet the full costs of optimal medical care, we shall have to settle for something less.

In the final analysis, the future of American medicine and, indeed, of world medicine will depend more upon limitations of man power and economy than upon the limitations of science. There is no better illustration of this fact than the one provided by the very disease which we have been considering. Were it possible merely to apply what is now known about diphtheria to every part of the world, this devastating malady could, for all practical purposes, be wiped from the face of the earth. Instead, however, it still rages in many lands. At the 1960 Asian Pediatric Conference, for example, a single Indian physician reported more than 2,000 cases of diphtheria. In the same year, only half this number was reported in the entire United States.

Modern medicine's basic predicament stems from the fact that "science tells us *how* to do things, but never tells us *what* to do among all the things that *could* be done." [14] What is done depends upon the decisions of society, made within the practical limitations of human and economic resources. These practical decisions will continue to determine the extent to which advances in medicine are applied to the benefits of mankind.

Where does this leave us, then? Progress in social organization has lagged far behind the technological advances of medical science. As a result, the full benefits of modern medicine are being received by only a minority. At the same time, there is an increasing awareness of their potentialities, and, as a result, there is more and more demand for better and less costly medical care. The greatest danger is that this demand will lead to hasty and drastic solutions, such as compulsory socialized medicine, which in the end would lower the incentive and quality of the medical profession and thus lead to suboptimal health service. Surely some sounder alternative can be found which will assure proper medical care to a greater proportion of the population and maintain the prestige of medicine at a level that will continue to attract talented and dedicated individuals to its ranks.

To arrive at such an alternative is the joint obligation of society and the medical profession. Neither can do the job alone, for the principal problems involved are combined socio-scientific ones which can be solved only by joint effort. If enough doctors abdicate their social responsibilities, medicine will inevitably become socialized. Conversely, if society leaves the matter entirely to the medical profession, service to the public may cease to be the primary objective of medicine.

The greatest deterrent to a satisfactory solution is faulty communication. In recent years, many physician groups have been accused of being insensitive to social needs. At the same time, large segments of the public are grossly ignorant of the problems which beset the modern doctor in an age of scientific revolution. Unfortunately, the medical profession has not yet learned how to communicate effectively with the public it serves. If its "social conscience" is as genuine as I believe it is, its leaders will intensify their efforts to become more articulate and to speak in a language which can be understood by the average layman. Only when the consequences of scientific progress, as typified by the story of diphtheria, are generally known will society give to the medical profession the kind of support it will have to have to bring to the majority of the people the full benefits of medical science.

SOURCE NOTES

MIASMAS

1. E. Caulfield, *The Throat Distemper of 1735–1740* (New Haven, Yale Journal of Biology and Medicine, 1939).
2. *Printed and Sold by S. Kneeland and T. Green, in Queenstreet, Over Against the Prison* (Boston, 1740).
3. *Kingston Church Records* (New Hampshire Genealogy Record, II, 43, III, 37).
4. J. Farmer and J. B. Moore, *Collections, Topographical, Historical and Biographical Relating Principally to New Hampshire* (1822), I, 143.
5. J. Fitch, *An Account of the Numbers that Have Died of The Distemper in the Throat within the Province of New Hampshire* (Boston, 1736).
6. *Journal of the Rev. Thomas Smith* (Portland, Me., 1894).
7. *Boston News-Letter* (Dec. 18-25, 1735).
8. *Boston News-Letter* (Feb. 19–26, 1736).
9. J. Fitch, *Two Sermons on Occasion of the Fatal Distemper Which Prevail'd in Sundry Towns within the Province of New Hampshire* (Boston, 1736).
10. Leviticus, 13: 45–46.
11. W. Eulloch, *The History of Bacteriology* (London, Oxford University Press, 1938).
12. H. Fracastorius, *De Contagione et Contagiosis Morbis et Curatione* (Venice, 1546), Vol. III. English translation by W. C. Wright (New York, G. P. Putnam's Sons, 1930).
13. W. Boghurst, *Loimographia, an Account of the Great Plague of London in the Year 1665*, ed. by J. F. Payne (London, 1894).

14. B. Cohen, *The Leeuwenhoek Letter* (Baltimore, Society of American Bacteriologists, 1937).

15. B. Marten, *A New Theory of Consumptions, More Especially of a Phthisis or Consumption of the Lungs* (London, 1720).

16. C. Linné, [Linnaeus], *Systema Naturae per Regna Tria Naturae* (12th ed., revised Holmiae, 1767), Vol. I, Part 2, p. 1326.

17. F. T. Lewis, "The Microscope in America," *Scientific Monthly*, LVII (1943), 249

18. F. W. Andrewes *et al.*, *Diphtheria, its Bacteriology, Pathology and Immunity* (London, His Majesty's Stationery Office, 1923).

19. Aretaeus, *The Extant Works of Aretaeus the Cappadocian*, edited and translated by Francis Adams (London, Sydenham Society, 1856).

20. Aetius, *Librorum Medicinalium Tomus Primus, Primi Scilicet Libri Octo Nunc Primum in Lucem Editi* (Venice, 1534), fol., Vol. VIII, p. 162 b.

21. A. H. Morejon, *Historia Bibliografica de la Medicina Española* (7 vols., Madrid, 1842–52).

22. J. de Villa-Real, *De Signis, Causis, Essentia, Prognostico et Curatione Morbi Suffocantis* (Compluti, 1611), Vol. II.

23. J. B. Cortesius, *Miscellaneorum Medicinalium Decades Denae* (Messina, 1625), fol., Part IX, letter 6, p. 696.

24. J. Chandler, *A Treatise of the Disease Called a Cold. . . . Also a Short Description of the Genuine Nature and Seat of the Putrid Sore Thoat* (London, 1761), Chapter IV, Sect. VI, p. 53.

25. F. Home, *An Inquiry into the Nature, Cause and Cure of the Croup* (Edinburgh, 1765).

26. P. Bretonneau, *Des Inflammation Spéciales du Tissu Muqueux et en Particulier de la Diphthérite ou Inflammation Pelliculaire Connue Sous le nom de Croup, de'angine Maligne, d'angine Gangréneuse* (Paris, 1826), 3 plates, 540 pp.

MICROBES

1. P. Bretonneau, *Traités de la Dothimenterie et de la Spécificité Publiés pour la Première fois d'après les Manuscrits Originaux avec un Avant-propos et des notes de L. Dubreuil-Chambardel* (Paris, Vigot, 1922), 368 pp.

2. A. Bassi, *Del Mal del Segno Calcinaccio o Moscardino, Mallattia che Affligge i Bachi de Seta e sul Modo di Liberarne li Bigatteje Anche le piu Infestate* (Lodi, 1835), Part I, Theory; (1836), Part II, Practice; (2d ed., Milan, 1837).

3. A. Bassi, *Sui Contagi in Generale e Specialmente su Quelli che Affligono l'umano Specie* (Lodi, 1844).

4. J. Snow, *On the Mode of Communication of Cholera* (2d ed., London, 1855), 162 pp.

5. W. Budd, *Typhoid Fever: Its Nature, Mode of Spreading, and Prevention* (London, 1873).

6. O. W. Holmes, *Puerperal Fever, as a Private Pestilence* (Boston, Tichnor and Fields, 1855).

7. I. Semmelweis, "Höchst Wichtige Erfahrungen über die Aetiologie der in Gebaranstalten Epidemischen Puerperalfieber," *Zeitschrift der k.-k. Gesellschaft der Aerzte zu Wien*, IV (1847), 242; V (1849), 64.

8. M. J. Oertel, "Experimentelle Untersuchungen über Diphtherie," *Deutsches Archiv für klinische Medizin*, VIII (1871), 242.

9. M. J. Oertel, *Die Pathogenese der Epidemischen Diphtherie. Nach Ihrer Histologischen Begründung* (Leipzig, 1887).

10. E. Klebs, "Beiträge zur Kenntniss der Pathogenen Schistomyceten," *Archiv für experimentelle Pathologie und Pharmakologie*, I (1875), 31.

11. E. Klebs, *Ueber Diphtherie* (Wiesbaden, Verhandlungen des Congresses für inner Medizin, 1883), p. 139.

12. R. Koch, "Die Aetiologie der Tuberculose," *Berliner klinische Wochenschrift*, XIX (1882), 221.

13. R. Koch, *Ueber die neuen Untersuchungsmethoden zum Nachweis der Mikrokosmen in Boden, Luft and Wasser* (Aerztliches Vereinsblatt für Deutschland, 1883), No. 237.

14. E. Löffler, "Untersuchungen über die Bedeutung der Mikroorganismen für die Entstehung der Diphtherie beim Menschen, bei der Taube und beim Kalbe," *Mitteilungen an dem k. Gesundheitsamt*, II (1884), 421.

15. E. Roux and A. Yersin, "Contribution à l'étude de la diphthérie," *Annales de l'Institut Pasteur*, II (1888), 629.

16. E. Roux and A. Yersin, "Contribution à l'étude de la diphthérie (2ᵉ memoire)," *Annales de l'Institut Pasteur*, III (1889) 273.

17. S. Kitasato, "Ueber den Tetanusbacillus," *Zeitschrift für Hygiene*, VII (1889), 225.

18. C. Fraenkel, "Untersuchungen über Bacteriengifte. II. Immunisirungsversuche bei Diphtherie," *Berliner klinische Wochenschrift*, XXVII (1890), 1133.

19. E. Behring and S. Kitasato, "Ueber das Zustandekommen der Diphtherie-Immunität und der Tetanus-Immunität bei Thieren," *Deutsche medizinische Wochenschrift*, XVI (1890), 1113.

20. E. Behring, "Untersuchungen über das Zustandekommen der Diphtherie-Immunität bei Theiren," *Deutsche medizinische Wochenschrift*, XVI (1890), 1145.

21. E. Wernicke, "Die Immunität bei Diphtherie," *Handbuch der pathologischen Mikroorganismen* (2d ed., von Kolle-Wassermann, 1913), Vol. V, p. 1011.

22. J. Fibiger, "Om Serumbehandling af Difteri," *Hospital-stidende*, VI (1898), 309, 337.

23. G. S. Wilson and A. A. Miles, *Topley and Wilson's Principles of Bacteriology and Immunity* (4th ed., Baltimore, The Williams and Wilkins Company, 1955), II, 1590.

24. T. Smith, "Active Immunity Produced by So-called Balanced or Neutral Mixtures of Diphtheria Toxin and Antitoxin," *Journal of Experimental Medicine*, XI (1909), 241.

25. E. Eehring, "Ueber ein neues Diphtherieschutzmittel," *Deutsche medizinische Wochenschrift*, XXXIX (1913), 873.

26. B. Schick, "Die Diphtherietoxin-Hautreaktion des Menschen als Vorprobe der Prophylaktischen Diphtherieheil-

seruminjektion," *Münchener medizinische Wochenschrift*, LX (1913), 2608.

27. G. Ramon, "Sur le pouvoir floculant et sur les proprietes immunisantes d'une toxine diphtherique rendue anatoxique (anatoxine)," *Comptes rendus de la Academie de sciences*, CLXXVII (1923), 1338.

28. F. M. Burnett, *Natural History of Disease* (New York, Cambridge University Press, 1959), Chapter XIX.

29. W. T. Russell, *The Epidemiology of Diphtheria During the Last Forty Years* (London, Medical Research Council, 1943), Special Report Series, No. 247.

30. J. S. Anderson *et al.*, "On the Existence of Two Forms of Diphtheria Bacillus—B. *diphtheriae gravis* and B. *diphtheriae mitis*—and a New Medium for Their Differentiation and for the Bacteriological Diagnosis of Diphtheria," *Journal of Pathology and Bacteriology*, XXXIV (1931), 667.

31. J. W. McLeod, "The Types, Mitis, Intermedium and Gravis of *Corynebacterium Diphtheriae*," *Bacteriological Reviews*, VII (1943), 1.

32. L. Barksdale *et al.*, "Virulence, Toxinogeny, and Lysogeny in *Corynebacterium Diphtheriae*," *Annals of the New York Academy of Science*, LXXXVIII (1960), 1093.

33. E. Caulfield, *The Throat Distemper of 1735–1740* (New Haven, Yale Journal of Biology and Medicine, 1939), p. 17.

MOLECULES

1. L. Barksdale *et al.*, "Virulence, Toxinogeny, and Lysogeny in *Corynebacterium Diphtheriae*," *Annals of the New York Academy of Science*, LXXXVIII (1960), 1097.

2. V. J. Freeman, "Studies on the Virulence of Bacteriophage-Infected Strains of *Corynebacterium Diphtheriae*," *Journal of Bacteriology*, LXI (1951), 675.

3. N. B. Groman, "Evidence for the Active Role of Bacteriophage in the Conversion of Non-toxigenic C. Diphtheriae to Toxin Production," *Journal of Bacteriology*, LXIX (1955), 9.

4. M. H. Adams, *Bacteriophages* (New York, Interscience Publishers, Inc., 1959).

5. W. Weidel, *Virus* (Ann Arbor, University of Michigan Press, 1959), p. 9.

6. A. M. Pappenheimer, Jr., in *Bacterial and Mycotic Infections*, ed. by René Dubos (Philadelphia, J. B. Lippincott Co., 1958), pp. 210-229.

7. C. G. Pope and M. Stevens, "Isolation of a Crystalline Protein from Highly Purified Diphtheria Toxin," *Lancet*, II (1953), 1190.

8. C. B. Anfinsen, *The Molecular Basis of Evolution* (New York, John Wiley & Sons, Inc., 1959).

9. S. F. Dudley, *The Schick Test, Diphtheria and Scarlet Fever* (London, Medical Research Council, 1923), Special Report Series, No. 75.

10. A. M. Pappenheimer, Jr., "The Diphtheria Toxin," *Scientific American*, XXXII (October, 1952).

11. A. M. Pappenheimer, Jr., in *Mechanisms of Microbial Pathogenicity* (New York, Cambridge University Press, 1955), pp. 40–56.

12. A. M. Pappenheimer, Jr., "Bacterial Toxins," *Federation Proceedings*, VI (1947), 479.

13. N. Strauss and E. D. Hendee, "The Effect of Diphtheria Toxin on the Metabolism of HeLa Cells," *Journal of Experimental Medicine*, CIX (1959), 145.

14. A. M. Pappenheimer, Jr., "Diphtheria Toxin. III. A Reinvestigation of the Effect of Iron on Toxin and Porphyrin Production," *Journal of Biological Chemistry*, CLXVII (1947), 251.

15. A. M. Pappenheimer, Jr., and E. D. Hendee, "Diphtheria Toxin. IV. The Iron Enzymes of *C. Diphtheriae* and Their Possible Relations to Diphtheria Toxin," *Journal of Biological Chemistry*, CLXXI (1947), 701.

16. A. M. Pappenheimer, Jr., and R. C. Williams, "Effects of Diphtheria Toxin on the Cecropia Silkworm," *Journal of General Physiology*, XXXV (1952), 727.

17. I. Kato and A. M. Pappenheimer, Jr., "An Early Effect of Diphtheria Toxin on the Metabolism of Mammalian Cells Growing in Culture," *Journal of Experimental Medicine*, CXII (1960), 329.

CONSEQUENCES

1. "The Crisis in American Medicine," *Harper's Magazine*, Vol. CCXXI, No. 1325 (October, 1960), p. 121.
2. M. B. Folsom, "Goals for the Nation's Health," an address given to the Southern Regional Education Board (Baltimore, August 6, 1960).
3. "U.S. Doctor Supply and Medical School Problems," New York *Times*, November 6, 1960.
4. "Physicians for a Growing America," Report of the Surgeon General's Consultant Group on Medical Education, Public Health Service (1959).
5. E. F. Potthoff, "The Future Supply of Medical Students in the United States," *Journal of Medical Education*, XXXV (1960), 223.
6. "Final Report of the Study Group on Mission and Organization of the Public Health Service," U.S. Government Printing Office (June 7, 1960), 0-553903.
7. C. P. Snow, *The Two Cultures and the Scientific Revolution*, The Rede Lecture (New York, Cambridge University Press, 1959), p. 5.
8. W. B. Wood, Jr., "The Underlying Cause of Unrest in University Medicine," *Journal of the American Medical Association*, CLXIV (1957), 548.
9. J. Barzun, *Teacher in America* (Boston, Little, Brown & Co., 1945).
10. W. B. Wood, Jr., "Teachers of Medicine," *Journal of Laboratory and Clinical Medicine*, XLI (1943), 6.
11. D. W. Atchley, "The Healer and the Scientist," *Saturday Review*, January 9, 1954.
12. D. W. Atchley, "The Changing Physician," *The Atlantic Monthly*, August, 1956.

13. W. B. Wood, Jr., in *The Choice of a Medical Career* (Philadelphia, J. B. Lippincott Co., 1961).
14. R. J. Dubos, in *The Great Issues of Conscience in Medicine*, The Dartmouth Convocation, Hanover, New Hampshire (September 8–10, 1960).